Trust Is Not Enough

Bringing Human Rights to Medicine

Trust Is Not Enough
Bringing Human Rights to Medicine

David J. Rothman
and
Sheila M. Rothman

Preface by Aryeh Neier

NEW YORK REVIEW BOOKS

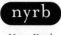

New York

THIS IS A NEW YORK REVIEW BOOK

PUBLISHED BY THE NEW YORK REVIEW OF BOOKS

TRUST IS NOT ENOUGH:
BRINGING HUMAN RIGHTS TO MEDICINE
by David J. Rothman & Sheila M. Rothman

Copyright © 2006 by David J. Rothman & Sheila M. Rothman

Preface © 2006 by Aryeh Neier

Copyright © 2006 by NYREV, Inc.

This edition published in 2006
in the United States of America by
The New York Review of Books
1755 Broadway
New York, NY 10019
www.nybooks.com

Library of Congress Cataloging-in-Publication Data

Rothman, David J.
    Trust is not enough : bringing human rights to medicine / by David J. and
Sheila M. Rothman ; preface by Aryeh Neier.
        p. ; cm. (New York Review Books collections)
    Includes bibliographical references and index.
    ISBN 1-59017-140-3 (alk. paper)
    1. Medical ethics. 2. Public health—Moral and ethical aspects. 3. Human rights—Health
aspects.
    [DNLM: 1. Bioethical Issues. 2. Human Rights Abuses. 3. Human Rights. 4.
Internationality. 5. Organ Transplantation—ethics. 6. Torture—ethics. 7. World Health.
WB 60 R846t 2006] I. Rothman, Sheila M. II. Title. III. New York Review Books collection.
R724.R626 2006
    174.2—dc22

                                                            2006002971

ISBN-10: 1-59017-140-3
ISBN-13: 978-1-59017-140-0
Printed in the United States of America on acid-free paper.
1 3 5 7 9 10 8 6 4 2

Contents

Preface

DAVID AND SHEILA ROTHMAN bring a distinctive voice to the discussion of medical issues. They are historians and the examination of historical background is a central factor in their thinking about contemporary developments. They are proponents of professionalism and, therefore, high standards; ethical principles and the engagement of the medical profession itself in maintaining those standards and principles also pervade their thoughts. And they are advocates of human rights. This makes them especially alert to abusive medical practices that may be condoned or even encouraged by repressive political regimes. Their commitment to human rights is reflected as well in their concern that patients should be able to obtain the information they need to make intelligent choices on matters that may involve life and death, and that medical professionals should strive, so far as is possible, to treat their patients fairly, respectfully, and appropriately.

The Rothmans' sensitivity to human rights is evident in their writings about such matters as human experimentation, the international traffic in human organs, and the ways that regimes such as those of the Romanian dictator Nicolae Ceauşescu and the Zimbabwean despot Robert Mugabe can have disastrous consequences for medical care. Concern for human rights also leads the Rothmans to be highly dubious of utilitarian solutions to questions about who is eligible for care that may be too costly to provide to all who need it. They are not persuaded by assertions about collective well-being nor by attempts to establish hierarchies that determine who is deserving of care. They avoid references to the whiff of eugenics in arguments for rationing heath care that view health not as an end in itself but only as a means to achieve other socially desirable ends. For them to point out that such arguments imply that some are "unworthy of life" would be too harsh, one understands, but their criticism of this approach to the rationing of health care is no less effective because of the evident restraint in their writing.

As the Rothmans indicate, I had a hand in enlisting them in two or three of the visits to far-off places where they looked into the connection between medical care and human rights. At the time, I was executive director of Human Rights Watch and I had discovered fairly early in my tenure there that, both for better and for worse, physicians had a significant role in dealing with abuses of human rights.

An episode that played an important part in my own thinking on such matters took place in 1981, soon after we established the Americas division of Human Rights Watch. On its behalf, I visited Chile that December. My visit was prompted by the arrest on December 10, at the conclusion of the annual Human Rights Day celebration,[1] of seven leaders of the Chilean Commission on Human Rights, a nongovernmental organization established to challenge abuses committed by the government of General Augusto Pinochet, who had seized power on September 11, 1973. When I got to Chile eight or nine days after the arrests, I learned that three of the seven men who had been detained had been tortured by the secret police—then known as the

---

1. December 10 is celebrated as Human Rights Day worldwide because it is the anniversary of the adoption of the Universal Declaration of Human Rights by the United Nations General Assembly in 1948.

DNI. By the time I arrived in Santiago, however, their interrogation, which took place while they were being tortured, had been completed. With no further interest in extracting information from them, the DNI had transferred them to a regular prison.

With the help of a well-connected official of the Chilean Commission on Human Rights who had served in two cabinet positions in the Christian Democratic government that preceded both Pinochet and the leftist president he overthrew, Salvador Allende, I got into the prison and managed to conduct interviews with two of the three men who had been tortured. (In those days, such flying visits by international human rights activists were not as frequent as they became a few years later and the Chilean government probably did not imagine that it needed to guard against such brazen intrusions.) One of the two torture victims I met seemed to have survived his ordeal reasonably well. The other was in bad shape so I spent most of the time I had in the prison talking to him.

When I saw Pablo Fuenzalida, it appeared to me that one side of his body was paralyzed. He told me that he had been strapped to a bedspring and given electric shocks to sensitive parts of his body. He thought this went on during parts of five days, though he was not really sure because he was blindfolded the entire time. He also told me that from time to time, he was examined by someone he thought was a doctor, who seemed to determine that he was capable of enduring additional electric shocks.

Following my visit to the prison, I went to the Foreign Ministry where I saw the director-general, the ministry's senior career officer. He vigorously denied that torture had taken place and later had a messenger deliver a packet to my hotel that contained photocopies of brief statements, apparently by physicians, which said that they had examined each of the seven men when they were transferred from the DNI to the regular prison and that all were in good condition. Though the statements were typed, the signatures that followed were indecipherable and there was no other information on the documents I received that identified the physicians.

I also paid a call on the Chilean Medical Society and saw that organization's president and a couple of his colleagues. When I complained that it appeared that Chilean physicians were participating in torture, they expressed dismay but none denied what I inferred from the evidence I had obtained nor seemed very surprised. Instead, they told me they believed they were helpless to act because not long after taking power, Pinochet had issued a decree stripping the country's professional associations of their authority to discipline their members. The government alone would exercise this power. I gave copies of the documents I had obtained with the illegible signatures to the Medical Society, but expected that nothing would come of this.

Somewhat later in the decade, the Chilean Medical Society did conduct investigations of complicity in torture by some physicians. As best I can tell, repugnance against such complicity was a factor in the eventual emergence of the Medical Society and its members as leaders in the effort to bring the Pinochet dictatorship to an end. In the process, many physicians took substantial risks. Though the actions of a few doctors who put their professional skills at the service of torturers were shameful, a great many more Chilean physicians conducted themselves honorably, providing care to torture victims and leading the struggle against a regime one of whose defining characteristics was its regular practice of torture.

Over time, my work at Human Rights Watch provided me with a host of examples of the positive part that physicians could play in the protection of human rights. Often they did so by reporting on the medical consequences of abuses. At other times, as when pathologists determined the causes of death, physicians had a crucial role in investigating abuses. Two examples from the 1980s, both involving the work of a then newly established group, Physicians for Human Rights, stand out in my thinking on this subject.

In 1988, at the end of the Iraq–Iran war, in which Saddam Hussein's forces had used chemical weapons to devastating effect against Iranian troops, reports circulated that he had turned such weapons against some of his own people, the Kurds in the town of Halabja. At the time, the Reagan administration supported Saddam Hussein because he was the enemy of America's enemy, Khomeini's Iran, and officials of the Department of Defense and the Central Intelligence Agency disputed the allegation that Saddam had used such weapons. (To his credit, Secretary of State George Shultz declined to go along with this whitewash.) It was not possible to get into Halabja to gather evidence at the site, but through physical examinations of survivors who had made their way across the Turkish border, and through interviews with them about what they had seen, a team of American physicians was able to determine that the allegations against Saddam's regime were indeed well warranted. (It is, of course, an historical irony that some of the same American officials who tried to clear Saddam Hussein of that charge in 1988 were prominent among those a decade and a half later who pointed to his use of chemical weapons at Halabja as evidence of his continuing possession of such weapons and his menace to the United States.)

The other example that stands out in my thinking about the investigative role of physicians involves the first Palestinian intifada, which occurred during the same period. A team of physicians who went to the occupied territories found that many Palestinians had suffered broken bones on the inside of their forearms. The physicians pointed out that if someone raised a forearm to ward off a blow during a melee, the bones susceptible to breakage would be those on the outside of the forearm. To break a bone on the inside of a forearm requires that a blow be administered while the person's arm is held down.

Another important way that physicians address human rights issues is by serving as advocates on behalf of the victims of abuses that have severe medical effects. Three of the five groups that came together to form the International Coalition to Ban Landmines in 1992, the group that was awarded the Nobel Peace Prize five years later, were substantially made up of physicians.[2] It did not require medical expertise to determine that landmines were responsible for maiming and killing thousands of civilians long after peace had supposedly been restored to lands ravaged by combat. Yet the participation of physicians in speaking out on such matters played an important part in calling attention to the gravity of this abuse and in lending a sense of urgency to the search for a solution.

In his capacity as president of the Institute on Medicine as a Profession, David Rothman has conducted training programs for physicians in advocacy. Yet the Rothmans are carefully nuanced in considering the most fundamental questions around which a certain amount of physician advocacy has been mobilized: Is there a right to health care, and if so, what kind of care, and how is this right to be enforced? The discussion of these issues in one of the essays published here focuses on South Africa, whose Constitutional Court has grappled with social and economic rights in particularly thoughtful decisions on the basis of the post-apartheid constitution, which goes further than that of any other country in attempting to provide guarantees for such rights. After reviewing the leading cases involving those issues brought before the South African court, the essay concludes that its decisions show "how fundamental principles such as the right to health care or housing need not be merely grandiose phrases. Rather, when appropriately defined and interpreted, such rights can set the standards that a government must aim to satisfy." Steering a course between disregard of assertions about such rights

---

2. The groups were Medico, a German organization; Handicap International, a French group; and Physicians for Human Rights. The other founders of the ICBL were Human Rights Watch and the Vietnam Veterans Foundation.

and efforts to impose rigid standards is, of course, where the difficulty lies. The South African approach to this question recognizes the tutelary role that courts may play within a democratic system. It recognizes that "the Constitutional Court cannot enforce such rights, but its decisions can provide leverage to advocacy groups, serve to educate the public, and force a hostile or indifferent government to act in ways that help bring greater dignity, freedom, and equality to its people."

This is at some remove from what is sought by many proponents of economic and social rights who imagine that a court is the place to force the other branches of government to accord them the benefits—health care, education, housing, employment—apparently guaranteed them by the Universal Declaration of Human Rights and by a number of international and regional treaties. They imagine that it is possible for a court to trump the political process in allocating a society's resources. In contrast, the Rothmans' vision here, like that of the South African Constitutional Court itself, though expressed differently, is more modest. Though the essay recognizes that courts lack the power to implement economic and social rights, as they can neither collect taxes nor require that funds be allocated to particular programs, it maintains that the judiciary can contribute effectively to the political process in which such questions must be resolved. Accordingly, when the Constitutional Court sided with the Treatment Action Campaign in the case requiring the government of South Africa to provide nevirapene to pregnant women to prevent mother-to-child transmission of HIV, it was not only acting as a check on irrational decision-making by a representative government. Another effect of the decision was to enhance the representativeness of that government by ensuring that those infected with HIV were heard in the political process. Judges, it is understood, have limited means to enforce their decisions. They depend on their ability to persuade the other branches of government not just of the correctness of their decisions but of their legitimacy and, thereby, to secure their cooperation in enforcement. When courts appear to go beyond the bounds of legitimacy and to make arbitrary and poorly justified rulings, as happened in the United States when the Supreme Court struck down New Deal legislation out of concern for the economic rights of property holders, they risk losing the ability to secure compliance. In matters involving a nation's purse as in questions about the use of its sword—both of which Alexander Hamilton, writing in the Federalist Papers, considered to be outside the scope of the judiciary—a court is, at the least, at the outer edge of the territory where it is perceived to enjoy legitimacy.

Though the essays published here were written over a period of nearly two decades, none of them is out of date. Some of the factual circumstances originally described by the Rothmans have changed— though many have not, and in other cases they have provided updates —but the questions of medical professionalism and human rights that they address in considering those circumstances are as timely today as when these essays first appeared. Bringing them together in one place allows one to see connections between them that were not apparent previously, making for a collection that is greater than the sum of its parts. Taken together, these essays present us with a picture of an ongoing struggle for the soul of a profession. Many of its members are as flawed and corruptible as the rest of us and because health care, at least in our own society, can be quite lucrative, many temptations may be put before them. Yet the calling that they pursue inspires some among them to adhere to a higher standard and provides critics such as the Rothmans with a basis for prodding their less scrupulous colleagues in that direction.

—Aryeh Neier
January 2006

Introduction

ALTHOUGH THE ESSAYS in this book recount different stories from different places at different times, they come together in their exploration of four major themes, each linking human rights and medicine. The first meeting point is their uncompromising commitment to the integrity of the human body. Under no circumstances should physicians be complicit in torture, beatings, or other cruel and unusual punishments. Furthermore, they should not participate in the plundering of body parts, no matter what rationale of medical need may be offered. The importance and meaning of these two principles inform the two case studies that open the book: the worldwide traffic in organs and the brutal system of punishment in India's prisons.

The second link between human rights and medicine is a commitment to informed consent and freedom from coercion. The idea is nowhere more forcefully expressed than in the Nuremberg Code, and human experimentation, therefore, is the focus for the next two essays. One examines research that was conducted in the United States, beginning with a study at Vanderbilt University between 1945 and 1948 in which pregnant women were fed radioactive iron; the other looks at human experimentation in developing countries, in particular the use of placebos in AIDS research.

The third uniting principle is a commitment to equity and fairness in the distribution of social resources and to the implementation of a just system for delivering health care. One essay looks at the especially difficult case of rationing scarce but potentially life-saving treatment, using Oregon's health care policies as a point of departure. The next addresses the more general question of a right to health. Many international bodies have proclaimed such a right, but is there a way to translate it into practice? The beginnings of an answer may well be found in the ways the South African Constitutional Court has interpreted the provisions for a right to health care in the nation's constitution, in order to expand access to medical treatment for a society living with the legacy of apartheid.

The final three essays address the most ancient principle of medical ethics—do no harm—and demonstrate its relevance for human rights. This violation of this principle helps the puzzle of why Romanian orphans in the Ceauşescu era contracted AIDS. It accounts for the harms done in Zimbabwe when whites tried to avoid desegregation by establishing their own private, for-profit hospitals. And it even has relevance to patient care in New York City, as revealed in the case of Libby Zion.

* * *

A word of explanation about the authorship of the essays. Chapter 3, 4, 5, and 9 were written by David Rothman; Chapters 1, 6, 7, and 8 were written by David Rothman and Sheila Rothman, and Chapter 2 was written by David Rothman with Aryeh Neier. All except Chapters 4 and 6 appeared in *The New York Review of Books* and have been revised and brought up to date for this book. Chapter 4 was originally delivered as the Fielding H. Garrison Lecture at the seventy-fifth annual meeting of the American Association for the History of Medicine, April 26, 2002, in Kansas City, Missouri; a revised version of the lecture appeared in the *Bulletin of the History of Medicine*, Vol. 77, No. 1 (Spring 2003). Chapter 6 was written especially for this book.

I

Bodily Integrity

I

THE INTERNATIONAL TRAFFIC
IN ORGANS

OVER THE PAST thirty years, transplanting human organs has become a standard and remarkably successful medical procedure, giving new life to thousands of people with failing hearts, kidneys, livers, and lungs. But very few countries have enough organs to meet patients' needs. In the United States, for example, some 80,000 people are on waiting lists for a transplant; 15 percent of patients who need a new heart will die before one becomes available.[1] The shortages are even more acute throughout the Middle East and Asia.

Since the mid-1990s and with the support of several organizations and foundations, we have monitored the global traffic in organs. In order to grasp fully how the system works, how shortages arouse desperation and reward greed, we have devoted particular attention to the trade in India, China, Thailand, Singapore, and the Philippines. As our account will demonstrate, would-be recipients are willing to travel nearly anywhere to get an organ and many surgeons, brokers, and government officials will do nearly anything to profit from the shortage.

The body part that accounts for most of the traffic is the kidney. Since the waiting list to obtain a kidney from a cadaver is very long, the best way to get one is from a living donor—usually from a sibling,

---

1. This data is from the OPTN/UNOS National Database, accessed November 25, 2005.

a spouse, a relative, or a friend. In the United States, living donation has become the source for more than half of all transplanted kidneys. But what if relatives are unwilling or unable to donate? Many people will then try to purchase a kidney.

The routes that they follow are well known to doctors and patients both by word of mouth and now, increasingly, through the Internet. Israelis travel to Belgium and have also been going to rural Turkey, bringing their surgeons along with them. South Africans use organs purchased in Brazil; Moldova and Estonia sell to Israelis, and Bulgaria and Romania sell to them and to other Eastern Europeans as well. Residents of the Gulf States, Egyptians, Malaysians, and Bangladeshis mainly go to India to take advantage of its flourishing market in organs. In the Pacific, Koreans, Japanese, and Taiwanese, along with the residents of Hong Kong and Singapore, fly to China where hospital officials profitably market organs of executed prisoners. The Philippines also has large numbers of kidneys available for purchase, and its hospitals actively try to sell them to the Japanese.[2] Overall, the international commerce in organs is unregulated, indeed anarchic. Just as we are being forced to assess the consequences of global financial markets for less-developed countries, so we must consider the effects of global markets in medical technologies and organs.

Although it is technically possible to pack kidneys in ice and send them by air between countries, the traffic is almost always in people, not organs. Part of the reason is that the country providing the kidney wants to collect the substantial hospital and surgical fees that come with transplantation. Part of the reason, too, is that health and hospital authorities in places like Japan or Israel would almost certainly refuse to transplant organs purchased and shipped from developing

---

2. David J. Rothman, "The Bellagio Task Force Report on Transplantation, Bodily Integrity and The International Traffic in Organs," *Transplant Proceedings*, Vol. 29, No. 6 (1997), pp. 2739–2745.

countries. They would have to defend publicly the ethics of such transactions—keeping them secret would be impossible—and risk the legal liabilities that could follow from using organs of unknown origin that might well be harboring deadly viruses.

No one we know of has calculated the size of the organ trade, but it probably amounts to several thousand transplants each year. Not only are shortages growing more acute but transplant technology has spread almost everywhere; as with other operations, when more surgeons are prepared to do a transplant, more patients will ask for one. Surgeons have also found that patients who receive an organ from a living donor have far better prospects than those who receive an organ from a cadaver. And transplant teams, wanting to satisfy their patients and remain competitive with rival groups, do not inquire into the sources of the organs that they use. They say they are surgeons, not detectives, and, besides, their only obligation is to the patient on the operating table.

Americans, for the most part, stay home, but wealthy foreigners come to the United States for transplants, and medical centers are permitted to allot 5 percent of their organs to them. Since such foreigners pay in cash, they have been known to go right to the top of the waiting list. In November 2005, the liver transplant program at St. Vincent's Medical Center in Los Angeles was decertified because surgeons had moved a Saudi national from fifty-second to first on the waiting list, bypassing patients who had been waiting longer and were more seriously ill. No one has said how much money changed hands but it could not have been a trivial amount.

Until the early 1980s and the discovery of the drug cyclosporine, transplantation had been a risky and experimental procedure, typically a last-ditch effort to stave off death. The problem was not the complexity of the surgery but the body's immune system, which attacked and rejected the new organ as though it were a foreign object. Cyclosporine moderated that response without suppressing the immune system's reactions to truly infectious agents. As a result, in countries with sophisticated medical programs, kidney and heart transplantation became widely used and highly successful procedures. More than 70 percent of heart transplant recipients were living four years later. Ninety-two percent of patients who received a kidney from a living donor were using that kidney one year later; 81 percent of the cases were doing so four years later, and in 40 to 50 percent of the cases, ten years later.

Transplantation spread quickly from developed to less-developed countries. By 1990, kidneys were being transplanted in nine Middle Eastern, six South American, two North African, and two sub-Saharan African countries. Kidney transplants are by far the most common, since kidneys are subject to disease from a variety of causes, including persistent high blood pressure, adult diabetes, nephritis (inflammation of vessels that filter blood), and infections, which are more usually found in poor countries. Most kidney donors can live normal lives with one kidney. (It is true that donors runs the risk that the remaining kidney will become diseased, but in developed countries, at least, this risk is small.) The transplant techniques, moreover, are relatively simple. Replacing one heart with another, for example, is made easier by the fact that the blood-carrying vessels that must be detached from the one organ and reattached to the other are large and relatively easy to handle. (A transplant surgeon once told us that if you can tie your shoes, you can transplant a heart.)

Fellowships in American surgical programs have enabled surgeons from throughout the world to master transplant techniques and bring them home. Countries such as India and Brazil built transplant centers when they might have been better advised to invest their medical resources in public health and primary care. For them the centers are a means for enhancing national prestige, for persuading their surgeons not to leave the country, and for meeting the needs of their own middle-class citizens.

Because of the spread of this technology, China now has more than fifty medical centers that perform kidney transplants, and in India hundreds of clinics are doing so. Reliable information on the success of these operations is hard to obtain, and there are reports that hepatitis and even AIDS have followed transplant operations. But according to physicians we have talked to whose patients have traveled to India or China for a transplant, and from published reports within these countries, some 70 to 75 percent of the transplants seem to have been successful.[3]

Most of the doctors and others involved in early transplants expected that organs would be readily donated as a gift of life from the dead, an exchange that cost the donor nothing and brought the recipient obvious benefits. However, it turns out that powerful cultural and religious taboos discourage donation, not only in countries with strong religious traditions but in more secular ones as well.[4]

In the Middle East, it is rare to obtain organs from cadavers. Islamic teachings emphasize the need to maintain the integrity of the body after death, and although some prominent religious leaders make an exception for transplants, others refuse. An intense debate occurred in Egypt when the government-appointed leader of the most important Sunni Muslim theological faculty endorsed transplantation as an act of altruism, saying that permitting it was to accept a small harm in order to avoid a greater harm—the same rationale that allows a Muslim to eat pork if he risks starvation. But other clerics immediately objected, and there is no agreement in favor of donation.

In Israel, Orthodox Jewish precepts define death exclusively as the

---

3. Xia Sui-sheng, "Organ Transplantation in China: Retrospect and Prospect," *Chinese Medical Journal*, Vol. 105 (1992), pp. 430–432.

4. *Organ Transplantation: Meanings and Realities*, edited by S. J. Younger, R. C. Fox, and L. J. O'Connell (University of Wisconsin Press, 1996).

failure of the heart to function, not as the cessation of brain activity, a standard that makes it almost impossible to retrieve organs. The primary purpose of statutes defining death as the absence of brain activity is to ensure that organs to be transplanted have been continuously supplied with oxygen and nutrients; in effect, the patient is declared dead, and a respirator keeps the heart pumping and the circulatory system working until the organs have been removed, whereupon the respirator is disconnected. Some rabbis give precedence to saving a life and would therefore accept the standard of brain death for transplantation. But overall rates of donation in Israel are very low. The major exceptions are kibbutz members, who tend to be community-minded, as well as more secular Jews.

In much of Asia, cultural antipathy toward the idea of brain death and, even more important, conceptions of the respect due to elders have practically eliminated organ transplantation from cadavers. For all its interest in new technology and its traditions of gift-giving, Japan has only a minuscule program, devoted almost exclusively to transplanting kidneys from living related donors. As the anthropologist Margaret Lock writes: "The idea of having a deceased relative whose body is not complete prior to burial or cremation is associated with misfortune, because in this situation suffering in the other world never terminates."[5]

For tradition-minded Japanese, moreover, death does not take place at a specific moment. The process of dying involves not only the heart and brain but the soul, and it is not complete until services have been held on the seventh and forty-ninth days after bodily death. It takes even longer to convert a deceased relative into an ancestor, all of which makes violating the integrity of the body for the sake of transplantation unacceptable.

---

5. "Deadly Disputes: Ideologies and Brain Death in Japan," in *Organ Transplantation: Meanings and Realities*, pp. 142–167.

Americans say they favor transplantation but turn out to be very reluctant to donate organs. Despite countless public education campaigns, organ donation checkoffs on drivers' licenses, and laws requiring health professionals to ask families to donate the organs of a deceased relative, the rates of donation are wholly inadequate to the need. As of November 2005, according to the United Network for Organ Sharing, nearly 68,000 people were awaiting a kidney transplant, 18,000 a liver transplant, and 3,100 a heart transplant. One recent study found that when families were asked by hospitals for permission to take an organ from a deceased relative, 53 percent flatly refused.

The literary critic Leslie Fiedler suggests that the unwillingness of Americans to donate organs reflects an underlying antipathy toward science and a fear of artificially creating life, a fear he finds exploited in the many Hollywood remakes of the Frankenstein story. Moreover, donation would force Americans to concede the finality of death, which Fiedler is convinced they are reluctant to do. We suspect, however, that the underlying causes are less psychological than social. Americans are unaccustomed to sharing resources of any kind when it comes to medicine. Since Americans refuse to care for one another in life—as witness the ongoing debacle of national health insurance—why would they do so in death? Receiving help is one thing, donating it is another.

If organs are in such short supply, how do other countries manage to fill the needs of foreigners? The answers vary. Belgium has a surplus of organs because it relies upon a "presumed consent" statute. Under its provisions, you must formally register your unwillingness to serve as a donor; otherwise, upon your death, physicians are free to transplant your organs. To object you must go to the town hall, make your preference known, and have your name registered on a national computer roster. When a death occurs, the hospital checks the computer base, and unless your name appears on it, surgeons may use your organs, notwithstanding your family's objections. We were told by health professionals in Belgium that many citizens privately fear that if they should ever need an organ and another patient simultaneously needs one as well, the surgeons will check the computer and give the organ to the one who did not refuse to be a donor. There is no evidence that surgeons actually do this; still many people feel it is better to be safe than sorry, so they do not register any objections.

One group of Belgian citizens, Antwerp's Orthodox Jews, has nonetheless announced they will not serve as donors, only as recipients, since they reject the concept of brain death. An intense, unresolved rabbinic debate has been taking place over the ethics of accepting but not giving organs. Should the Jewish community forswear accepting organs? Should Jews ask to be placed at the bottom of the waiting list? Or should the Jewish community change its position so as to reduce the prospect of fierce hostility or even persecution?

Because its system of presumed consent has worked so well, Belgium has a surplus of organs and will provide them to foreigners. However, it will not export them, say, to Milan or Tel Aviv, which would be entirely feasible. Instead, it requires that patients in need of a transplant come to Belgium, which then benefits from the surgical fees paid to doctors and hospitals.

India has an abundant supply of kidneys because physicians and brokers bring together the desperately poor and the desperately ill. The sellers include impoverished villagers, slum dwellers, power-loom operators, manual laborers, and daughters with small dowries. The buyers come from Egypt, Kuwait, Oman, and other Gulf States, and from India's enormous middle class (which numbers at least 200 million). They readily pay between $2,500 and $4,000 for a kidney (of which the donor, if he is not cheated, will receive between $1,000 and $1,500) and perhaps twice that for the surgery. From the perspective of most patients with end-stage renal disease, there is no other choice.

For largely cultural reasons, hardly any organs are available from cadavers, dialysis centers are scarce and often a source of infection, and only a few people are able to administer dialysis to themselves at home (as is also the case in the US). Thus it is not surprising that a flourishing transplant business has emerged in such cities as Bangalore, Bombay, and Madras.

In 1994, perhaps for reasons of principle or because of public embarrassment, a number of Indian states, including the regions of Bangalore, Bombay, and Madras, outlawed the practice, which until then had been entirely legal. But the laws have an egregious loophole so that sales continue almost uninterrupted. A detailed and persuasive report in *Frontline*, one of India's leading news magazines, explained how the new system works.[6] The legislation permits donations from persons unrelated to the recipient if the donations are for reasons of "affection or attachment" and if they are approved by "authorization committees." These conditions are easily met. Brokers and buyers coach the "donors" on what to say to the committee—that he is, for example, a cousin and that he has a (staged) photograph of a family gathering to prove it, or that he is a close friend and bears great affection for the potential recipient. Exposing these fictions would be simple enough, but many committees immediately approve them, unwilling to block transactions that bring large sums to hospitals, surgeons, and brokers.

Accurate statistics on kidney transplantation in India are not available, but *Frontline* estimates that about one third of transplants come from living, unrelated donors; four years after the new law went into effect, the rate of transplantation returned to its earlier levels. It is true that not every hospital participates in the charade, that the market in kidneys is less visible than it was, and it may well be that fewer foreigners are coming to India for a transplant. But the lower classes

6. "Kidneys for Sale," *Frontline*, Vol. 14 (December 13–26, 1997), pp. 64–79.

and castes in India, already vulnerable to so many other abuses, continue to sell their organs.

China is at the center of the Pacific routes to organ transplantation because it has adopted the tactic of harvesting the organs of executed prisoners. In 1984, immediately after cyclosporine became available, the government issued a document entitled "Rules Concerning the Utilization of Corpses or Organs from the Corpses of Executed Prisoners." Kept confidential, the new law provided that organs from executed prisoners could be used for transplants if the prisoner agreed, if the family agreed, or if no one came to claim the body. (Robin Munro, then of Human Rights Watch/Asia, brought the law to light.) That the law lacks an ethical basis according to China's own values is apparent from its stipulations. "The use of corpses or organs of executed prisoners must be kept strictly secret," it stated, "and attention must be paid to avoiding negative repercussions." The cars used to retrieve organs from the execution grounds cannot bear health department insignia; the people involved in obtaining organs are not permitted to wear white uniforms. In our own interviews with Chinese transplant surgeons, none would admit to the practice; when we showed them copies of the law, they shrugged and said it was news to them.

But it is well known to other Asian doctors. Physicians in Japan, Hong Kong, Singapore, and Taiwan, among other countries, serve as travel agents, directing their patients to hospitals in Wuhan, Beijing, and Shanghai. The system is relatively efficient. Foreigners do not have to wait days or weeks for an organ to be made available; executions can be timed to meet market needs and the supply is more than adequate. China keeps its exact number of executions secret, but Amnesty International calculates on the basis of executions reported in newspapers that there are at least 4,500 a year, and perhaps three to four times that many. Several years ago a heart transplant surgeon told us that he had just been invited to China to perform a transplant; accustomed to long waiting periods in America, he asked how he could be certain that a heart would be available when he arrived. His would-be hosts told him they would schedule an execution to fit his travel schedule. He turned down the invitation.

China's system also has its defenders. Why waste the organs? Why deprive prisoners of the opportunity to do a final act of goodness? The objections should be obvious. The idea that a prisoner on death row—which in China is often a miserable hovel in a local jail—can give informed consent to his donation is absurd. Moreover, there is no way of ensuring that the need for organs might not influence courtroom verdicts. A defendant's guilt may be unclear, but if he has a long criminal record, why not condemn him so that a worthy citizen might live?

To have physicians retrieve human organs at an execution, moreover, subverts the ethical integrity of the medical profession. There are almost no reliable eyewitness accounts of Chinese practices, but Taiwan has also authorized transplants of organs from executed prisoners and its procedures are probably duplicated in China. Immediately before the execution, the physician sedates the prisoner and then inserts both a breathing tube in his lungs and a catheter in one of his veins. The prisoner is then executed with a bullet to his head; the physician immediately moves to stem the blood flow, attaches a respirator to the breathing tube, and injects drugs into the catheter so as to increase blood pressure and cardiac output. With the organs thus maintained, the body is transported to a hospital where the donor is waiting and the surgery is performed. The physicians have become intimate participants in the executions; instead of protecting life, they are manipulating the consequences of death.

The motive for all such practices is money. The Europeans, Middle Easterners, and Asians who travel to China, India, Belgium, and other countries pay handsomely and in hard currencies for their new organs. Depending on the organization of the particular health care system and the level of corruption, their fees will enrich surgeons or medical centers, or both. Many of the surgeons we interviewed were quite frank about how important the income from transplants was to their hospitals; with their governments now appropriating less than 10 percent of hospital budgets, the need for outside revenues was clear. The physicians, of course, were far more reluctant to say how much of it they kept for themselves. Still, a leading transplant surgeon in Russia is well known for his vast estate and passion for horses. His peers in India and China may be less ostentatious but not necessarily less rich. They will all claim to be doing good, rescuing patients from near death.

The international trade in organs has convinced many of the poor, particularly in South America, that they or their children are at risk of being mutilated and murdered. Stories are often told of foreigners who arrive in a village, survey the scene, kidnap and murder several children, remove their organs for sale abroad, and leave the dissected corpses exposed in the graveyard.[7] In Guatemala in 1993 precisely such fears were responsible for one innocent American woman tourist being jailed for a month and another being beaten to death.

Villagers' anxieties are shared by a number of outside observers who believe that people are being murdered for their organs. The author of the report of a transplant committee of the European Parliament unequivocally asserted:

> Organized trafficking in organs exists in the same way as trafficking in drugs. It involved killing people to remove organs

---

7. This and other examples of lending credence to the rumors may be found in the United States Information Agency Report of December 1994, *The Child Organ Trafficking Rumor*, written by Todd Leventhal.

which can be sold at a profit. To deny the existence of such trafficking is comparable to denying the existence of ovens and gas chambers during the last war.

So, too, the rapporteur of a UN committee on child welfare circulated a questionnaire asserting that "the sale of children is mainly carried out for the purpose of organ transplantation." It then asked: "To what extent and in what ways and forms do these violations of children's rights exist in your country? Please describe."[8]

The stories of organ-snatching have an American version. We have heard it from our students, read about it on e-mail, been told about it with great conviction by a Moscow surgeon, and been asked about it by more than a dozen journalists. According to the standard account, a young man meets an attractive woman in a neighborhood bar; they have a few drinks and go back to her place, whereupon he passes out and then wakes up the next morning. In some versions, he has a wound on his side and when he seeks medical attention, he learns that he is missing a kidney. In other versions, he wakes up in a tub filled with ice, and a message scrawled on the mirror in lipstick says: Call 911 or die.

Although there have been sporadically reported stories of robberies of kidneys from people in India, we have not found a single documented case of abduction, mutilation, or murder for organs, whether in North or South America. By chance we were in Guatemala when the atrocities of 1993 are alleged to have occurred, and heard seemingly reliable people say there was convincing evidence for them. We stayed long enough to see every claim against the two American women tourists proven false. Nevertheless, the villagers' fears and accusations are understandable in the light of their everyday experience. The bodies of the poor are ordinarily treated so contemptuously

---

8. V. Muntarbhorn, *Sale of Children: Report of the Special Rapporteur to the United Nations Commission on Human Rights*, January 12, 1993.

that organ-snatching does not seem out of character. In Guatemala, babies are regularly kidnapped for sale abroad in the adoption market. Local doctors and health workers admitted to us that "fattening houses" have been set up so that kidnapped babies would be more attractive for adoption.

But it is extremely dangerous to investigate the adoption racket, since highly placed officials in the government and military take a cut of the large sums of money involved. Moreover, if street children in Brazil can be brazenly murdered without recrimination, it is not far-fetched for slum dwellers to believe that the organs of the poor are being removed for sale abroad. And since girls and boys can be kidnapped with impunity to satisfy an international sex market, why not believe they are also kidnapped to satisfy an international organ market?

In truth, medical realities make such kidnappings and murder highly unlikely. The rural villages and the urban apartments in which they are alleged to secretly take place do not have the sterile environment necessary to remove or implant an organ. Organs from children are too small to be used in adults. And however rapacious health care workers may seem, highly trained and medically sophisticated teams of surgeons, operating room nurses, anesthesiologists, and technicians are not likely to conspire to murder for organs or accept them off the street. Had they done so, at least one incident would have come to light during the past twenty years.

As in all other Asian countries, families in Thailand are unwilling to donate an organ from a deceased relative. The country has a very high rate of traffic deaths—the result of widespread alcoholism, drug use, and a large number of motorcycles and motorbikes, called put-puts, driven by riders who do not wear helmets. But few organs become available for transplantation because Thais, whether for religious reasons or because of popular superstition, will not allow surgeons to remove them before cremation. The waiting list for a transplant is long, and because many of the people waiting are relatively well off, hospitals and surgeons are in a position to make substantial profits. The Thai health care system is made up of a network of public hospitals and private, profit-seeking hospitals. Since the public hospitals are generally overcrowded, uncomfortable, and unreliable, people who can afford it use for-profit hospitals. They are modern, clean, well equipped, and staffed with skilled physicians. In fact, the staff physicians, along with some administrators, are the major stockholders in the hospital corporation and are eager to make profits. Thus the hospitals have successfully promoted themselves as centers for medical tourism. Europeans use them for cosmetic surgery or dental work at prices that are 50 to 75 percent lower than at home. (At the same time, many Thais, as well as Europeans and Americans, come to Bangkok in search of easily available, low-cost sex, frequently supplied by prostitutes; AIDS has spread widely.) For the same reasons, some, but by no means all, of the hospitals have entered the kidney trade.

Selling organs, we found, can be highly profitable. Some private hospitals are unwilling to admit accident victims on the grounds that they are too poor to pay for an extended stay with complicated procedures. But their more aggressive competitors make a different calculation. If they admit traffic victims who then die, and if their families are willing to donate their organs, the hospital would then have two kidneys available for transplant into two patients able to afford the $10,000 cost of an operation that would cost about $100,000 in the US. This was precisely the calculation that was made by Siroj Kanjanapanchapol, chief transplant surgeon and head of Bangkok's Vachiraprakarn General Hospital (VGH).

Siroj had VGH admit a young pregnant woman who was in a coma following an auto accident and had been taken at first to a rural hospital. Siroj persuaded the family to agree that she be transferred to

VGH, promising that they would not be charged for the cost of care. He also had them sign a consent form authorizing the removal of her kidneys if she died. Following her death, Siroj gave them a $2,500 payment for "funeral expenses." He removed her kidneys, transplanted them into two patients, and charged each of them not only for the surgery but for the full amount of the "gift" to the family. Thus, for an expenditure of $2,500, Siroj and VGH made $25,000.

Siroj and three of his hospital colleagues came under investigation, probably because they had quarreled with another VGH administrator, who described what happened to the Thai Legal Association, the *Bangkok Post*, and the Thai Medical Council, which set up an inquiry. One of the witnesses from the hospital said the patient had not been officially brain dead when her organs were removed. Siroj and his colleagues were accused of unethical medical conduct and were indicted for murder, the first such case in Thailand.[9]

Siroj, when we talked to him, vigorously defended himself. There was nothing wrong, he said, with rewarding the family's willingness to donate the organs by waiving their medical charges at the hospital. And there was nothing wrong with allowing the patients who received the organs to reward the donors for their noble act. As for charges that the patient was still alive, Siroj claimed that it was too cumbersome to obtain the required three signatures certifying brain death—surely two, which is in fact the standard in most countries, was enough—and he had obtained the signatures of two colleagues.

The Thai Medical Council carefully investigated the case. It discovered that VGH has consistently violated the laws banning commerce in organs. The hospital regularly transplanted kidneys from

---

9. It is not the first such prosecution elsewhere. Until a few years ago, the Japanese refused to recognize brain death; the first surgeons to perform a heart transplant in Japan were charged with murder, as was a heart transplant recipient who had the procedure done abroad. None of them was convicted.

living donors who were neither blood relatives nor spouses of the recipients. VGH also paid out substantial sums to families for agreeing to a donation, and then charged the two recipients of the organs the full cost of the payment. It even bribed people in other hospitals to transfer patients near death to VGH and paid ambulance drivers to bring badly injured patients to its emergency room. The Medical Council, moreover, concluded that Siroj, along with other transplant surgeons, frequently ignored the criteria for establishing brain death. The transplant surgeon, who because of possible conflict of interest was not supposed to certify brain death, often did so. For all these reasons, the Medical Council resolved to punish Dr. Siroj "in the most serious way and without mercy" and rescinded his medical license. His trial on the murder charge was postponed several times but finally, in February 2005, the criminal court acquitted him of murder, ruling that the patients had died before their kidneys were removed.

Because Thailand has active medical and legal authorities, the illicit transplant activities came to light and at least some of them have been stopped. Most of the poorer countries, however, lack the professional and civic organizations that might oppose commerce in organs. Thailand is also different in having a respected monarchy. The Queen publicly endorsed the efforts of the Thai Red Cross to oversee the distribution of organs for transplantation. Over the past several years, the Thai Red Cross has been trying to improve the regulation of transplantation. It established an Organ Donation Committee (ODC), which has the authority to distribute cadaveric organs and to license transplant centers. As a very careful and thorough Thai government review concluded in 2003, the regulatory framework now operating is "adequate." However, it also identified glaring weaknesses. The ODC is a small organization with limited funding and it has a very conservative attitude. Although it can request relevant documents from transplant centers to ensure transparency and compliance with rules and regulations, it rarely exercises this power, fearful that tough regulation will make medical centers reluctant to perform the operations. In the end, surgeons and administrators are not as free as they once were to cut their own deals with families and would-be donors, but profiteering in organs remains a distinct possibility.

Singapore's government, unlike its neighbors, carefully regulates organ distribution and has successfully avoided financial corruption. But its system suffers from something else: a fundamental bias that effectively excludes Muslims from getting transplants.

Singapore's citizens, like other Asians, object to organs being removed from deceased relatives; as a result, the waiting list for kidneys is long. Singapore has an extensive network of dialysis centers; most people—61 percent—pay for treatment themselves, but the rest get government assistance. Still, many patients need transplants and so they travel to China to get the organs of executed prisoners; indeed, a handful of them, ten to fifteen a year, get organs from prisoners who are executed in Singapore. As surgeons explained to us, capital punishment is carried out in Singapore by hanging; the moment the trapdoor swings open and the neck is snapped, orderlies take the body to an adjoining operating room to have the organs removed. However, neither travel nor executions have much of an effect on the waiting list.

In 1987, Singapore enacted the Human Organ Transplantation Act (HOTA), a law unique in Asia. Anyone who suffers a fatal accident is presumed to be a kidney donor, unless he or she had formally "opted out" of the system by signing a card that declares, "I hereby object to the removal of my kidneys upon my death for transplantation," and then sending it to the Organ Donor Registry. To avoid provoking public protests, the act included two qualifications. It restricted the presumed consent to road accidents; terminally ill patients and their families would not have to worry that hospital physicians were neglecting them in order to obtain their kidneys.

HOTA, moreover, only applied to kidneys, not to the heart, which is considered by Singapore families the most precious organ. The number of donations from cadavers still varies from year to year but it now averages forty, not, as before, fewer than ten. The law, however, excluded all Muslims, including the ethnic Malays who make up some 15 percent of Singapore's population. Although Muslim religious leaders, like Orthodox Jewish rabbis, disagree among themselves on whether organ donation is permissible, Muslims generally are reluctant to donate organs. Still, it was not cultural pluralism but political discrimination that accounted for Singapore's exclusion of Muslims from receiving transplants.

In typical bureaucratic Singaporean style, the policy on transplants is written, codified, and available for all to see. We were given a copy at our first interview. An elaborate point system governs the national transplant waiting list. Patients have to accumulate some forty to fifty points to reach the top of the list and receive an organ. Medical criteria count, and so does severity of illness. Each year on the waiting list brings the would-be recipient 2.5 points. Social criteria are even more important. Full-time professional employment brings five points, full-time ordinary employment, four points. Age matters as well: people under thirty-one receive five points, and no one over sixty is eligible for transplant.

Muslims go on the list with a debit of sixty points. Since they have a record of opting out of the donor pool, the government argues they should be penalized. But no one else in Singapore who opts out is treated this way. It is true the debit is canceled if the would-be recipient agrees to donate his organs after death, and if, in addition, two Muslim friends also sign such a donation agreement. In effect, this concession is no concession at all but amounts to a demand for heretical behavior or conversion: abandon Muslim principles or forgo a transplant.

Anti-Muslim bias pervades Singaporean policies generally. Relatively few Muslims hold public office or high military positions. The government apparently believes that Muslims are more loyal to Islam than to Singapore and fears what might happen if a conflict erupted with Malaysia. But in another sense, the bias in medical treatment runs even deeper. No other country we know of has penalized persons who don't consent to contribute their organs when they die. When we asked transplant surgeons about the exclusion of Muslims, we were told bluntly that Singapore has its own standards. To the best of our knowledge, no organization, no transplant society, and no international medical group has protested this blatant discrimination.

Lying outside Manila's small district of office buildings and hotels are its vast and wretched slums. The pollution is thick there, the stench of garbage strong. The Philippines was for fifty years an American colony and the US, which supported the repressive and incompetent Marcos regime, bears a heavy responsibility for such misery.

Many Filipinos understandably seek to emigrate. Young women study nursing so that they can find jobs in US hospitals. As soon as medical students graduate, many of them take the examinations administered at the American embassy that will allow them to practice in the US. The numbers are so large that an American embassy official thought that Philippine medical schools required their students to pass the American test. Not surprisingly, a great many slum dwellers in Manila are ready to sell their kidneys.

Kidney disease, it turns out, occupies a special place in the history of the Philippines because Ferdinand Marcos suffered from it. He had his own collection of dialysis machines; when dialysis failed, he had two kidney transplants. (The surgeons, we were told, were flown in from the United States.) Marcos built the most impressive medical facility in Manila, the National Kidney and Transplant Institute (NKTI). It remains the leading public transplant center in the country, performing more transplants than any other hospital, public or private.

Where do the kidneys they transplant come from? In fact, they are sold openly and legally. Physicians and state officials readily defend sales of kidneys, citing the views of "ethicists" on the faculty of a local Catholic college to the effect that selling one's organs should be seen as a matter of free choice. Many residents of a squatter community called Tondo, which is located on the top of a garbage dump, have sold their kidneys. In 1999, an enterprising Manila television reporter filmed an hour-long program on the local kidney trade, including scenes in which row after row of men from Tondo lifted their shirts to show the camera the long and jagged scars from operations to remove kidneys.

As the men explained, and the physicians that we interviewed confirmed, medical teams go out to the slum, perform blood and tissue tests on the men, store the results, and then, when a would-be recipient arrives for a transplant, they get in touch, sometimes through a broker of organs, with the man whose blood and tissue provide the best match for a transplant. When asked about their health, the men complained of a variety of pains and disabilities. When asked about their economic condition, many of them said they were worse off. Before they sold their kidneys, they had typically worked at loading ships on the docks. After the sale, they were no longer physically able to do the heavy lifting required, or they had been summarily fired because their bosses thought they were no longer able to do it.

The television program and subsequent press stories forced government and hospital officials to defend their policies. Almost every one of them insisted that nothing was wrong with people selling kidneys; the only problem was with the middlemen, the brokers, who were exploiting the sellers. The traffic in organs, they said, merely had to be regulated, not ended. But the principles and methods proposed for regulation were so flimsy as to demonstrate unequivocally that the only concern was to maintain a profitable business. The formula the officials proposed to govern the transactions would regulate nothing. According to the chief surgeon of the NKTI and a colleague from a local Catholic college, the sums to be paid to the sellers should not be so large as to be "irresistible," or so small as to be "exploitative." But why would anyone sell a kidney unless the money seemed irresistible? And the practice in itself is exploitative.

None of our questions seemed to trouble the politicians, surgeons, hospital administrators, and academics we talked to. When we asked Juan Flavier, a former minister of health now in the Philippine Senate, whether he was concerned that Philippine practices violated World Medical Association (WMA) principles, he said that to the best of his knowledge, the WMA did not vote in the Philippines. When we asked a Catholic college faculty member how he could argue in favor of organ sales when the Pope had issued an injunction against it, he expressed surprise that the Pope had taken such a position. When we asked surgeons how they felt about violating the policies of international transplant societies, they told us that dialysis was in such short supply in the Philippines and kidney donation so rare that only the sale of kidneys could save their patients from death. And when we asked whether such patients were a small elite, limited to those able to afford the purchase of a kidney, the surgery, and lifetime costs of anti-rejection drugs, we were told that yes, this was mostly true, but after all, the Philippines was a very poor country.

Some degree of national shame seems to have prompted the government in 2003 to enact an Anti-Trafficking in Persons law. But the statute is most interesting for what it omits rather than what it includes. Section 4 declares: "It shall be unlawful for any person . . . to recruit, hire . . . transport or abduct a person by means of threat or use of force, fraud, deceit, violence, coercion, or intimidation for the purpose of removal of organs of said person." But apparently it is still perfectly acceptable to buy an organ from a slum dweller, while holding to the claim that the contract was voluntary and no force or coercion was involved.

*   *   *

It is not the abuses of organ trafficking but the shortage of organs that is the chief concern of many bioethicists and economists as well as transplant teams and patients. A number of them have been urging a reconsideration of the principle that organs should not be bought and sold. It is not an easy proposition to defend: practically every international medical body has condemned the idea of a market in organs and none has revised its position. The declaration of the WMA (a statement which we helped formulate) unequivocally outlaws traffic and sale of organs. Basing its policy on the principle of "free and informed decision-making," the WMA resolved:

> Payment for organs and tissues for donation and transplantation should be prohibited. A financial incentive compromises the voluntariness of the choice.... Organs suspected to have been obtained through commercial transaction should not be accepted for transplantation.[10]

It also insists that because prisoners are not in a position "to give consent freely and can be subject to coercion," the organs of prisoners "must not be used for transplantation."

Moreover, in direct response to evidence of a flourishing trade in kidneys in Eastern Europe, the parliamentary assembly of the Council of Europe issued a declaration in 2003 on "trafficking in organs." The assembly insisted that "this type of crime should not remain the sole responsibility of countries in Eastern Europe," that the press and television should not be the only ones to investigate it, and, still more notably, that physicians and others who participate in such activities should face criminal penalties. It urged all member states to tighten

---

10. "World Medical Association Statement on Human Organ and Tissue Donation and Transplantation," adopted by the 52nd WMA General Assembly in Edinburgh, Scotland, October 2000.

their laws on the donation of organs and to establish "the legal responsibility of the medical profession for tracking irregularities and sharing information." Criminal codes should be amended "to insure that those responsible for organ trafficking are adequately punished, including sanctions for...brokers, intermediaries, hospital/nursing staff and medical laboratory technicians," along with "medical staff who encourage and provide information on 'transplant tourism.'" The assembly encouraged member states "to deny national medical insurance reimbursements for illegal transplants abroad" and to "deny national insurance payments for follow-up care of illicit transplants."

Nevertheless, marketplace solutions are attracting unprecedented levels of support and gaining respectability. If only markets were allowed in kidneys, it is claimed, then the shortage would shrink, even disappear. As one transplant surgeon put it: "Discussing organ sales simply does not feel right, but letting candidates die on the waiting list [when this could be prevented] does not feel right either."[11]

The argument most frequently made to justify the ethics of kidney sales is that the sellers are entitled to exercise autonomy and, if they chose to sell, they would personally benefit; the sums they would receive would improve their life chances. One group of American physicians, bioethicists, and social scientists declares that kidney sales should be allowed, since "we cannot improve matters by removing the best option that poverty has left."[12] The bioethicist Robert Veatch has recently adopted this position, dropping his longstanding opposition to sales. His position is that because we are and will continue to be so uncaring and neglectful of the well-being of the poor, it is wrong to stand in the way of the one measure that would help them. But of

---

11. A. Matas, "The Case for Living Kidney Sales: Rationale, Objections and Concerns," *American Journal of Transplantation*, Vol. 4 (2004), pp. 2007–2017.

12. R. Veatch, "Why Liberals Should Accept Financial Incentives for Organ Procurement," *Kennedy Institute of Ethics Journal*, Vol. 1 (2003), pp. 19–36.

course, the question is whether it actually would help them—or would it introduce still more deleterious effects?

The information that has accumulated on the growing trade in organs completely contradicts the claim that sale would enable the poor to escape from poverty. An anthropologist from Berkeley, Lawrence Cohen, has interviewed thirty families from Madras with a relative who sold a kidney; another team, based at Pennsylvania State University, surveyed some three hundred people in Madras who had sold a kidney six years earlier. Both came to the identical conclusion: the people who sell kidneys are generally in debt before they sell a kidney and back in debt after they sell. "Decisions to sell a kidney," the team concluded, "appear to have less to do with raising cash toward some current or future goal than with paying off a high interest debt to local moneylenders. Sellers are frequently back in debt within a few years."[13]

Cohen goes even further, suggesting that once a geographic region becomes known to organ brokers as a likely source of kidneys, the brokers intensify their search for sellers there; creditors then become more aggressive in calling in debts, and relatives of patients become still more reluctant to donate a kidney when they can buy one. In other words, the result is a wider market in organs. As Amartya Sen has persuasively argued, economic development is too easily thwarted by notions of a "false liberty," the kind implicit in a so-called right to sell a kidney. Such practices deflect attention from the changes that are necessary to modernize an economy. Escaping from poverty requires fundamental changes in a country's economy, not incentives for the poor to sell their body parts.[14]

---

13. L. Cohen, "Where It Hurts: Indian Material for an Ethics of Organ Transplantation," *Daedalus*, Vol. 128, No. 4 (Fall 1999), pp. 135–165; M. Goyal, "Economic and Health Consequences of Selling a Kidney in India," *Journal of the American Medical Association*, Vol. 288 (2002), pp. 1589–1593.

14. D. J. Rothman, "Ethical and Social Consequences of Selling a Kidney," *Journal of the American Medical Association*, Vol. 288 (2002), pp. 1640–1641.

* * *

Is there anything that might be done to curtail the trade in organs? Although the major national and international medical bodies do oppose the sale of organs and the transplantation of organs from executed prisoners, none has been willing or able to to move beyond rhetoric and take action to enforce their views. The WMA in 1984, 1987, and 1994 condemned "the purchase and sale of human organs for transplantation." But the WMA only provides "guidance to medical associations, physicians, and other health care providers"; it neither has nor seeks authority to discipline organizations or practitioners and has adopted no measures of its own. It leaves it to national medical societies to "severely discipline the physicians involved." One WMA official did tell us that when China requested admission to the association, the WMA made it a condition that China agree to hold an international conference on the ethics of organ transplantation, particularly the use of executed prisoners. China agreed, and was admitted to the WMA, whereupon it postponed the promised conference indefinitely. The WMA has done nothing by way of reaction.

The World Health Organization has also begun paying attention to organ transplantation, convening experts and issuing policy statements. In May 2004, it called for "national oversight" of organ transplantation and "measures to protect the poorest and vulnerable groups from 'transplant tourism' and the sale of tissues and organs, including attention to the wider problem of international trafficking in human tissues and organs." But like the Council of Europe, whose opposition to trafficking we noted earlier, the WHO lacks powers of enforcement and the ability to implement such programs. Both organizations can only urge member states to take action.

It is, therefore, all the more discouraging to note that national medical organizations, a few exceptions aside, have not taken up the challenge. In 2002, the British General Medical Council banned from practice Dr. Bhaget Makkar, a general practitioner who, in a taped interview with an undercover reporter, declared that in return for payment, he could arrange for a living donor in the UK or in India. But imagine what might happen if medical bodies took proclaimed principles seriously, if they established a permanent monitoring body and kept close surveillance on organ donation practices. What if they threatened to withhold training fellowships from countries which tolerated exploitative practices, and did not accept Indian, Singaporean, or Filipino surgical residents? What if they refused to hold international meetings in those countries, and, as was the case with South Africa under apartheid, did not allow physicians from those countries to attend their meetings? What if they put pressure on drug companies such as Novartis, the manufacturer of cyclosporine, to sell their product only to doctors and hospitals that meet strict standards in obtaining organs? Medicine has become such a global enterprise that the doctors in those countries would not tolerate such sanctions and might well work successfully to change national practices. But as with the organs themselves, the willingness to use the moral authority of medicine as a force for change has, so far, been in short supply.

We can only hope that the medical profession, on its own or in response to external pressures, will begin to take its social and ethical responsibilities seriously and promote a universal commitment—one that could be enforced—to preserving the integrity of the bodies of all citizens. So far there is little sign that the medical profession is willing to accept any such obligation.

2

INDIA'S AWFUL PRISONS

INDIA HAS STRONG claims to being the world's largest democracy. It holds elections and regularly replaces one governing party with another. Its press is exceptionally outspoken and its judiciary, especially in the higher courts, is aggressively independent. Moreover, a variety of private and government agencies promote social welfare not only through traditional relief activities but by bringing lawsuits on behalf of the poor.

Nevertheless, if one believes that a democracy should include a system of checks and balances, formal or informal, that would prevent the government from acting lawlessly, India fails. This failure was apparent in the early years of the separatist agitation in the Punjab and Kashmir. By official count, 3,212 civilians—apart from armed militants and the troops fighting them—were killed in 1990 during the Indian government's campaign to crush these movements. Many believed the totals were much higher and that at least in Kashmir most of the victims died at the hands of the armed forces and the police. Although the subsequent cease-fire between India and Pakistan reduced the level of violence, serious abuses continue; suspects are detained for long periods and accusations of torture abound. Moreover, the government's response to the violence committed on Muslims by Hindu fundamentalists has been feeble, with perpetrators rarely brought to justice. In all, India's behavior is a highly dramatic demonstration of how the government fails to exercise restraint in enforcing the law.

In 1991, with these concerns to mind, Aryeh Neier, then head of Human Rights Watch, and I went to India. Human Rights Watch had just initiated a series of investigations of prisons in different countries, including the US, and we agreed to take the assignment to India. The country had long interested both of us—I had previously served a six-month stint as Fulbright Lecturer in Delhi—and we were convinced that conditions of incarceration were an apt indicator of a government's commitment to fairness and to restraints on arbitrary authority. They also revealed the degree of respect a government had for the principle of bodily integrity. In fact, abuse and torture became the focal point of our investigation and subsequent report, thus linking our work on prisons to one of the central issues in human rights and medicine.

What we found in India was that violations by government officials were flagrant and commonplace. In the major cities anyone unlucky enough to be arrested and jailed faced a far greater likelihood of torture and physical abuse than in many other countries that lacked India's democratic institutions. We anticipated that detainees and prisoners would be badly treated to some degree, if only because life was harsh for many law-abiding Indians. What dismayed us, however, was the extent of the brutality to which most prisoners were subjected.

In India an official commitment to egalitarianism is taken for granted, to the point that an intense debate over civil rights typically addresses the extent to which special benefits should be given to untouchables and other "backward castes." But egalitarianism, somewhat to our surprise, had no place in criminal justice. The system was explicitly biased in favor of the more prosperous classes. Prisons, for example, gave special privileges to virtually all upper- and middle-class inmates, even if they had committed extremely violent crimes. Even more unexpected was the fact that prisoners who were guilty of violent political offenses were in some respects treated as an elite group. They had, among other things, a more varied and ample diet than other prisoners and they could read books and articles that were denied to the others.

According to Indian law, every person who is arrested and held in custody must be brought before a magistrate within twenty-four hours of arrest. If the magistrate does not issue an order authorizing the prisoner to be held for up to fourteen days, he or she must be set free, and under no circumstances can the police hold a suspect without trial for more than ninety days. In practice, however, except for the fortunate few who could afford to hire a lawyer and put up bail, prisoners were often kept in jail without trial for weeks or months. In some cases, the police evaded the twenty-four-hour rule by not immediately recording an arrest. In many more cases, judges signed orders that prisoners continue to be held in custody without even requiring that they appear in court and without setting any time limits, even after weeks and months had passed.

People arrested were in the greatest physical danger when they were held in local police jails, where they were usually kept in crowded cells with only the most rudimentary sanitation facilities. Torture was commonplace. Experienced lawyers told us that more than half the people arrested in Bombay and an even higher proportion of those arrested in New Delhi were subjected to the "third degree"—a term commonly used in India to describe heavy beatings and other practices that could be described as torture.

Shortly before our arrival, one of India's most dynamic civil liberties groups, the People's Union for Democratic Rights (PUDR) in New Delhi (which remains very active today), published a report on people who had died while in police custody: almost all of them came to its attention through newspaper accounts. (India has a number of local civil liberties organizations but with a few exceptions, budgets are tiny, staffs are composed of volunteers, and their impact on criminal justice issues is limited.) By these means, the PUDR estimated that forty-eight people, typically under the age of thirty, died in police lockups in Delhi between 1980 and 1989. "Most of these people," the PUDR said, "died due to severe beating and prolonged torture. Practically every person taken to a police station in connection with some or the other offense in our country is subjected to severe beating and torture.... Sticks, boots and belts and wooden rollers are the most common instruments of beating. Sexual abuse, designed not only to hurt but also to humiliate, is part of the torture. Naked or seminaked men are a common sight in police lockups." Torture, it concluded, was "regular and systematic, whose end product is sometimes death."

Other Indian civil liberties groups issued similar reports. In 1988, twenty people died in police custody in Andhra Pradesh; fifteen in Bihar; eight in Kerala; twenty-two in Uttar Pradesh; and nineteen in West Bengal. The claims by officials that some of the prisoners had been drunk or ill, or had committed suicide, could not be supported by medical evidence since it was almost unheard-of for medical representatives of the family or of independent agencies to be allowed to participate in an autopsy. To complicate matters further, the Hindu practice of cremation often made independent autopsies impossible when doubts were raised about the causes of death. Under these circumstances, the evidence could not be conclusive, but it appeared that each year throughout India at least several hundred people died after being tortured. A deputy inspector general of police, Shailendra Misra, concluded:

> The brutal behavior of our police is established beyond doubt ... [in the] police commissions, surveys of public opinion and reports on specific instances of brutality.[1]

---

1. Shailendra Misra, *Police Brutality: Analysis of Police Behavior* (New Delhi: Vikas Publishing House, 1986), p. 44. The book is a revised version of a dissertation by Mr. Misra, a longtime professional police officer, written for the Indian Institute of Public Administration.

For women the greatest danger of police detention was rape. The National Expert Committee on Women Prisoners, whose chairman was the retired Supreme Court judge Krishna Iyer, reported that only six institutions throughout the country were exclusively for women, and their inmates were serving long-term sentences. Fewer than 20 percent of women in pretrial detention were in a separate prison; everywhere else they were in mixed prisons, mainly in separate wings or cells but, as the Iyer commission found, always under the authority of male guards.

How often did guards sexually exploit the women, most of whom were migrants from rural areas and lacked the protection that family or community connections could provide? Answers were particularly difficult to obtain, for in India, to an even greater extent than in Western countries, victims risk punishment or ostracism if it becomes known that they have been raped. If they are married, they are likely to be abandoned by their husbands and families, and if they are single, their chances of marriage are virtually lost. Thus rape is seldom reported, and when it happens to women in police custody, the silence is all the greater. Even if the victim were able to accuse her assailants, it is almost certain that she would suffer more than they would. The only clues to what happens come from incidents uncovered more or less by chance. The Delhi police themselves recently acknowledged that between 1988 and 1990 there were fourteen rapes of women in custody, and twenty-four police officers were named as responsible. Suspensions and dismissals followed, but so far as we could find, none of the twenty-four officers was convicted of a crime.

No doubt some police mistreated the people in their custody in order to force them to confess and plead guilty, thereby making their work easier and improving their reputation for efficiency. But these motives should not be given much weight. According to Indian law, confessions made before a judge are inadmissible at trial; in that respect, Indian defendants are better protected than they would be in the United States, where the Miranda rules only entitle suspects to be warned about their rights and not to be questioned without a lawyer present if they so choose. But the Indian rule is less protective than it seems, because evidence obtained as a result of a confession to the police, such as stolen property, can be used in court. Still, if the crime does not involve property, the value of a confession diminishes.

Moreover, if the police simply wanted a conviction they would have little reason to beat up and abuse, for example, poor rural migrants who took trains to the city without paying the fare. In most such cases, the person arrested has no ticket and there is no need to coerce a confession. The police are also frequently called to deal with cases of assault involving people who know each other; here, too, beatings to obtain a confession are unnecessary—the victim and neighbors would testify to what happened—but they occur anyway.

Why, then, so much violation of bodily integrity? It turned out that police torture in India had a long history. In 1854, when the British governor of Madras established a commission "for the Investigation of Alleged Cases of Torture," it received almost two thousand complaints. The commission concluded that torture was a standard practice and gave gruesome details:

> Among the principal tortures in vogue in police cases we find the following: twisting a rope tightly around the entire arm or leg so as to impede circulation; lifting up' by the moustache; suspending by arms while tied behind the back; searing with hot irons; placing scratching insects, such as the carpenter beetle, on the navel, scrotum and other sensitive parts; dipping in wells and rivers, till the party is half suffocated; squeezing the testicles; beating with sticks; prevention of sleep; nipping the flesh with pincers; putting pepper or red chilies in the eyes or introducing them into the private parts of men or women; these

cruelties occasionally persevered until death sooner or later ensues.[2]

Since this report was issued, many other commissions—some national, others sponsored by state governments—have made similar findings. The report of Inspector Misra, who served as director of a national police commission between 1977 and 1980, concluded that "the current methodology of third degree does not show any remarkable refinement over the methods described by the Torture Commission of 1854."[3]

Police brutality continued to flourish, we found, largely because of widespread corruption. Policemen had low status in India and were poorly paid; as with many other Indian officials they felt driven to supplement their incomes. The detainees themselves, or their families, were threatened with torture if they did not bribe the police—a threat that could work only if those who do not pay, or cannot pay, were in fact tortured. As Misra and the police commission observed:

> With a policeman the reputation for expert brutality fetches more money than actual brutality, but of course the reputation has to have a solid foundation. Once a policeman acquires a reputation for expert third degree he makes enormous quantities of money in daily crime work by simply withholding his customary brutality.[4]

In such a system people with money or connections could usually find a way to avoid being tortured, while virtually the only people subjected to severe police brutality were from the lowest classes and

2. Torture Commission Report, April 16, 1855, paragraph 67.

3. Misra, *Police Brutality*, p. 32.

4. Misra, *Police Brutality*, pp. 62–63.

castes. Since they had little political influence, the issue of police brutality was mostly ignored in Indian political life.

At the same time, we were frequently told, middle-class people, who almost always were spared brutal punishment, tended to believe that it was the most effective method for deterring crime. A report by a West Bengal civil liberties group on people killed in custody found that "to everyone it appears quite natural that the police should beat up any arrested person." As in other countries where police brutality took place as a matter of course—Brazil, with its police death squads, was an extreme example—the wide acceptance of torture reflected a lack of faith in the legal criminal justice system. Illegal methods flourished partly because the legal ones seemed inadequate.

In fact, India did not appear to suffer from soaring crime rates. No one placed much confidence in the government's statistics on crime, but academic experts who analyzed the crime rates were convinced that the streets in Delhi or Calcutta were relatively safe, and most visitors would agree. In India, as elsewhere, probably the most reliable crime statistics are for murder, one of the few crimes that are universally reported. In 1986, the most recent year for which we could obtain data, there were 27,269 murders and another 4,195 criminal homicides, a combined total lower than that for the United States, although India's population was three and a half times larger.

But whatever the rate of crime, and whatever the findings of commissions and civil liberties organizations, there were no administrative or legislative groups organized to check or discourage police brutality. In a society teeming with slums and desperate poverty, many people believed that the only sure way to maintain order was to have the police act first and ask questions later. That the police were notoriously corrupt themselves contributed to the public's willingness to tolerate police brutality. After all, some people said, if the culprits had not been beaten, it would have meant that the police had accepted their bribes.

Tradition and custom shaped life in prison as well. More than forty years after the end of British rule, the prisons were still technically governed by the Prisons Act of 1894. Since prison officials were anxious to avoid being held accountable, however, the various state prison manuals based on the 1894 law were collectors' items, not only in short supply but expensive as well. (We bought a copy of the Punjab manual in a Delhi bookstore for twenty dollars, and were repeatedly told how lucky we were to find one.) A number of commissions have attempted to update and revise the code, but except in a few states, Indian state parliaments have not enacted new legislation. The mostly unread authoritative text remained the 1894 act.

Not only the regulations but the day-to-day reality of India's prisons seemed archaic. In fact, the use of prisons, which in the West grew swiftly with modernization, had not become widespread in India; imprisonment was probably not more extensive then than it was under British rule. The most thorough investigation of the prisons, the All India Committee on Jail Reform (whose chairman was the retired Supreme Court justice Anand Mulla), found that there were 1,220 prison facilities in the country as of December 31, 1980, of which 822 (67 percent) were police jails, while almost all of the others were state prisons; together they held some 160,000 inmates; more recent estimates put the figure at 184,000. Well over half of these inmates were awaiting trial. In view of the inaccuracy of the records in some Indian states, these figures may have been too low; but if there were as many as 250,000 prisoners in a population of 850 million, the incarceration rate would be 29 per 100,000. In the United States, the incarceration rate per 100,000 was 426, in the Netherlands, 40.

Such low rates would have been cause for satisfaction in India if they did not also reflect the extent of police brutality. When the police tortured unconvicted offenders and then let them go or even killed them, imprisonment became superfluous. If the number of inmates was low, it was partly because many people were not tried but were punished by brutal treatment. Often we could find no clear reason why one person was beaten or tortured and sent home while another was beaten and kept in prison. Petty offenders made up about half of the prisoners serving time; the others had committed felonies such as robbery and assault, or worse. About a third of the convicted inmates served less than a year, 23 percent served between one and ten years, and the rest (44 percent) ten years or longer.

The All India Committee observed that many of the inmates came from the "underprivileged sections of society," noting that "persons who have means and influence generally manage to remain beyond the reach of the law even if they are involved in violation of the law." The extent to which low-caste Indians were imprisoned also emerged from a study of the prisons of the state of Orissa. Situated on the northeast coast of India, Orissa's population of more than twenty million had roughly the same proportion of urban and rural residents as the entire country. The tribes and castes that were "scheduled," that is, declared legally to be victims of discrimination and in need of protection, accounted for almost two thirds of the prisoners—about four times their proportion in India.[5] By comparison, black men accounted for 43 percent of the inmates in prisons and jails in the United States, also about four times their proportion in the population.

But there the comparison ended. India still followed the standards of the 1894 act by categorizing prisoners according to their social class. (A similar system prevailed in other countries of the Indian subcontinent, among them Pakistan, which shared the British colonial legacy.) Inmates classified as A or B were persons who by social status, education, and habit of life had been accustomed to a superior mode of living. Habitual prisoners could be included in this class by

---

5. Samarendra Mohanty, *Crimes and Criminals: A Socio-economic Survey* (New Delhi: Ashish Publishing House, 1990), pp. 72–77.

order of the inspector general of prisons. Category C consisted of "prisoners who are not classified in class A and B." People of higher classes and castes—those with property or from socially superior families or who had education—thus were set apart from the poor, the educated, and the low caste. It was not what you had done (which in the United States determined whether you were sent to a minimum, medium, or maximum security prison) or how you behaved in prison, but who you were that counted.

The classifications made a huge difference to a prisoner's life. A state investigation of the prisons of Tamil Nadu (the relatively progressive province that includes Madras) reported, matter-of-factly, that the daily allotment for feeding class A and B prisoners ranged from fourteen to seventeen rupees (around one dollar), while for C prisoners it was seven to eight rupees. The A and B prisoners were allowed to buy fruit and other food of "good nutritive value"; the others were not. The privileged prisoners were allowed to write and receive one letter a week; the others, one letter every two weeks. A and B prisoners could receive any newspapers; the others only those on a prescribed list. In still other jurisdictions, the A prisoners were exempted from menial labor and from such restraints as handcuffs and irons, all of which were standard for C-class prisoners.

The classification system increased the authority—and the corruption—of prison administrators. The official regulations provided that state officials classify the inmates, but in fact the prison administrators did so. The power to decide each prisoner's grade and privileges increased their control over the prison population and their ability to exchange favors for money. Inmates with money were usually prepared to pay the going rate for A or B status, and although hard evidence of such payoffs was not easy to find, every student of Indian prisons we knew of, whether inside or outside the system, agreed that such corruption was rampant. At the same time long-term convicts—that is, hardened criminals—were formally assigned most of the duties ordinarily performed by American prison guards. They were in a position to hand out or deny favors and to extract payment for them. Even if there were no payoffs, a prisoner's wealth and status would usually decide his classification. Relatively well-off prisoners could also hire lawyers who would devote themselves to seeing to it that their clients were accorded a privileged status.

Almost every aspect of a prisoner's life, we found, was determined by his ability to pay. In the Tihar jail in New Delhi, which held between five thousand and eight thousand prisoners, more than 90 percent of the inmates were in class C. We were not allowed to enter the jail, despite repeated requests to do so, but reliable sources told us that most of the prisoners lived in barracks, slept on the floor, worked in the prison factory for a paltry wage that was generally not paid, and were fed two small loaves of bread twice a day, along with some lentils and very small portions of vegetables. Inmates who had some money would buy—usually from guards, sometimes from inmates—a bed for the night or week, or a better work assignment. Since the diet was hardly adequate for survival, they bought food at the prison canteen or bribed the kitchen staff. If they had no money, they would try to win favors from better-off inmates by running errands for them, washing their clothes, or performing sexual services.

The system, as a former prisoner put it, also "makes the doctor a king." He could, for a price, recommend a special diet—milk, eggs, meat—or get a prisoner some time off by prescribing him a few days in the prison hospital. It was never much of a hospital—there was hardly any medical treatment in the prisons—but it was better than standard C conditions. To the best of our knowledge, no Indian medical society had protested these conditions and individual physicians seemed more content to manipulate the system to their own financial benefit rather than expose it.

Conditions for most women prisoners were almost equally harsh. The investigating committee headed by Justice Krishna Iyer of the

National Supreme Court found that the six special institutions for women were "better than other custodial centres although hardly adequate." In the mixed institutions, "clothing, work, education, or even medical examination were generally not available," and there were "no beds, bedsheets or pillows, just a cane mat." "Human rights cannot survive in such jails," the committee concluded, and this statement applied to virtually all the penal institutions in India.

Virtually the only groups that had condemned the abuses and corruption of the criminal justice system were civil liberties organizations, but they had not had much effect. They conducted investigations of the deaths of the people who were in custody, and the lawyers who volunteered their services were dedicated; but they had no national organization, no professional staff members, and depended entirely on volunteers who do civil rights work at home or at their regular business offices. As one student of the human rights movement in India observed, these organizations tended to become active when there was a crisis—for example a series of deaths in a local prison—and then "they fade away, even die out, only to resurface, often in a new form at the time of another crisis."[6] It was almost impossible for them to conduct the sustained campaigns that would be required to expose and stop such practices as police torture or to reform the prison system.

By contrast, virtually every country in Latin America and the Caribbean had one or more human rights organization with its own offices and professional staff. (The exceptions were Cuba, where the Castro regime has made this impossible, and some of the smaller Caribbean nations.) That India should lag behind these countries might seem surprising because efforts to defend civil liberties there went back to 1936, when Jawaharlal Nehru established the national Indian Civil Liberties Union, which was active until independence

---

6. Smitu Kothari and Harsh Sethi, *Rethinking Human Rights* (Delhi: Lokayan, 1989), p. 178.

was declared in 1947. (Rabindranath Tagore was its honorary president and Krishna B. Menon was its first secretary.) After Nehru became prime minister he wrote a letter to his fellow members recommending that the ICLU be dissolved, apparently believing that his government could be counted upon to protect civil liberties. The ICLU soon ceased to exist.

A new civil liberties movement was organized in India in 1975 when Nehru's daughter, Prime Minister Indira Gandhi, imposed a state of emergency and jailed several thousand political opponents. To resist her repressive policies, a longtime associate of Nehru and Gandhi, Jayaprakash Narayan, founded the People's Union for Civil Liberties and Democratic Rights. The new group became less active in 1977 when Mrs. Gandhi was defeated at the polls, and many of its members went into the Janata government. By 1980, the movement split into two groups: the People's Union for Civil Liberties, which concentrates on protecting existing constitutional rights, and the People's Union for Democratic Rights, which seeks broader reforms of Indian society. The two groups have collaborated at times, particularly in investigating and denouncing the failure of the police to protect the Sikhs in 1984 when some three thousand of them were murdered in Delhi after Mrs. Gandhi's assassination.

The Indian civil liberties movement was mainly concerned with the need to defend peaceful dissenters from repression; but for most of the period since independence, peaceful dissenters had been able to make their views known, while much of the current opposition in Punjab and Kashmir has condoned violence, and such anarchist-minded groups as the Naxalites have been committed to the violent overthrow of the government.

In India, moreover, the representatives of civil liberties groups that we met, unlike their counterparts elsewhere in the world, were invariably hostile to the idea of obtaining support from foreign donors such as the Ford Foundation, the Dutch and German Foundations, the

European Community, or church groups such as Oxfam. While civil rights leaders badly needed the funds such organizations could be willing to contribute, they said they feared that outsiders would impose their own concerns, and the Indian organizations would be seen as manipulated by foreign interests. The outright rejection—really disdain—for foreign assistance that we encountered in India had no counterpart in any other country we knew of; it seemed to reflect a more general antagonism toward anything that smacked of Western involvement in India's social affairs. Indian leaders frequently recalled to us the case of the Asia Foundation, which provided financial support for many Indian institutions and claimed to be wholly independent of the US government but was revealed in the late 1960s to be a conduit for CIA funds. That some Indian organizations were shown to have been duped at the time made other foreign agencies suspect.

The prospects for social reform in India appeared to us to be dim; we had little optimism about reforming criminal justice. Since no powerful political constituencies were much concerned about police activities or prison corruption, and since the middle and upper classes had no personal stake in change and many people were persuaded that the current system worked reasonably well, the Indian human rights movement seemed the only force that could bring about reforms. When some of the movement's leaders asked us, as outsiders, for our views on what might be done, we observed that because the prison system was relatively manageable in size, change could be accomplished without spending large amounts of money. Were the case otherwise, the prospect of reform would be unrelievedly bleak. Indeed, we proposed that significant improvements could be accomplished through relatively inexpensive administrative reforms that were entirely consistent with the prevailing ideology (although not the practice) of the Indian government and the leading political parties.

Clearly the prisoner classification system should be eliminated, not only for reasons of fairness but to make the conditions of the prisons a more urgent concern of people from the middle classes. So long as the "haves" could buy their way out, the "have nots" would be left to suffer the system's worst abuses. It could be argued that abolishing the A and B classes would only serve to make the standards of class C life more pervasive; the leveling could be downward, not upward. Nevertheless, the risk should be taken, for there seemed no other way to broaden awareness of police and prison practices.

Second, while corruption is never easy to weed out, it was so extensive among police and prison officials that even a limited effort to bring some honesty and accountability to the system would be telling. A few firings and prosecutions might work wonders.

Third, to curtail the abuses in police detention, the practice of turning over arrested people to police custody after they are arraigned before magistrates should be eliminated. The practice amounted to a judicial invitation to the police to use torture and, in the case of women, to engage in rape. It would be difficult to enforce the rule that an arrested person be arraigned within twenty-four hours, since the police were the ones who counted the time; but once offenders were brought before a judge, the courts could release many more of them on bail or personal recognizance. If they must be held in custody to ensure they won't run away, they should be placed in facilities under court supervision, not in police lockups.

Moreover, the prosecution of police who abused detainees might deter others. It would cost little to require that independent doctors, not police doctors, conduct postmortem examinations. And were families and reform organizations given access to these findings, still another deterrent to abuse would be provided.

Finally, ways should be found to strengthen the civil liberties and human rights organizations in India. In view of their fears of foreign funding and foreign interference, suggestions from outsiders would automatically be suspect; but if the Indian organizations themselves devised new strategies for promoting human rights, they would find their counterparts in the United States and Europe eager to help them.

The original publication of our findings had an unanticipated consequence, which has made it more difficult to analyze what, if anything, has changed in India's prison system. It had not seemed worth mentioning at the time that both Aryeh and I had been questioned by Indian security police before we left the country. When I handed the woman at the airline check-in counter my ticket and passport, she examined it, checked her computer, made a call, and in a moment, a security official was at my side asking me to follow him. We went to a nearby small, windowless room, where he and two colleagues proceeded to question me about the visit, where we had traveled, with whom we had met. The questioning was polite and my apparent inability to recall names did not provoke hostility; when I noted that I had met with a Mr. Singh, the Indian equivalent of Smith, my questioners merely chuckled. After some forty-five minutes, I looked at my watch, suggested it was time for me to make my flight, no one objected, and I was on my way. I stopped to call Aryeh at his hotel and alert him to the incident, and he would later, back in New York, tell me that the security police came to his hotel early the next morning and asked the same questions in the same manner. We both agreed that they seemed most interested in whether we had been to Kashmir and would be writing about detention, torture, and killings there. When it became clear that our primary focus was more on the jail and prison system, they lost interest.

But there was a repercussion. Since that time, I have requested a visa from the Indian embassy three times, and have been refused each time. An acquaintance who works in the US embassy in Delhi tried to intervene on my behalf but was not successful; he told me that my name is engraved on the "do not allow back" list. The Indian ambassador to the US leaned in as well, to no avail. Clearly, the story we wrote touched a sensitive chord. The Indian government does not take criticism lightly.

Unable to return and see for myself what has or has not changed in the Indian system of incarceration, I rely on other people's research. Happily, the materials are thorough, persuasive, and consistent. Sadly, our description of conditions does not require much revision.

The Prison Act of 1894 is still the prevailing law and several efforts to update it have failed. The number of prisons in the country (1,119) has not changed at all. Overcrowding persists: while official capacity is 229,713, occupancy stands at 313,635—136 percent of capacity. As the absolute numbers suggest, the rate of incarceration remains very low. According to the Sentencing Project, a remarkably thorough research and advocacy organization, India's rate is 29 per 100,000 of the population. The next lowest country is Japan (58); the US is at the top (726), followed by Russia (532) and South Africa (413). But again, the incarceration rate in India goes hand in hand with beatings and abuse. The UN's special rapporteur on torture has declared that the practice of torture on persons in police custody in India is "endemic." The US State Department's Country Reports on Human Rights Practices (2004) also comments on the frequency with which authorities use torture during interrogations either to get information or to extort money, the continuing problem of rape of women inmates, and the unacceptably high death rate of those in custody. The State Department also cites extraordinary overcrowding (New Dehli's Tihar jail held four times more prisoners than its capacity) and a paucity of food and medical care. Amnesty International has issued similar findings. One of its reports focused on the city of Ahmedabad, where scores of Muslims were detained in jails in the aftermath of communal conflict and the killing of fifty-nine Hindus. The detentions were often illegal and the treatment brutal.

In 1993, India established a National Human Rights Commission, and prison practices, including torture and death in pre-trial detention facilities, take a prominent place on its agenda. The NHRC collects data and publicizes abuses, but it has not been effective in bringing about change or pinpointing responsibility. It remains understaffed and dependent on the government (whose officials it is supposed to investigate) for its funding. It receives an extraordinary number of complaints from putative victims of abuse each year, between 60,000 and 70,000. The result is an enormous backlog and an ongoing inability to successfully prosecute cases or penalize people it believes culpable. The consulting company of McKinsey even performed an analysis, pro bono, of how it might do its job more efficiently, but even the NHRC admits its own inadequacies.

Reading its annual report is dismaying. In 2002–2003, of 82,231 cases it disposed of, there were 263 "disappearances," 3,595 illegal detentions and arrests, 706 instances of violence to inmates, 689 rapes, 434 related to prisoner harassment, 44 cases of lack of medical facilities in jails, 9,622 complaints of "other police excesses," and on and on. One can only imagine how many other cases were never reported to it. Indeed, why anyone would bother to bring a complaint before it is puzzling. In 2002–2003, it directed disciplinary action/prosecutions in just five cases and asked for compensation in another thirty-nine.

The NHRC did attempt to draft a revision of the 1894 Prison Act but its efforts went nowhere. It urged the Indian government to sign the 1984 Convention Against Torture and Other Cruel, Inhuman or Degrading Treatment or Punishment, but met no success. India is still not a party to the convention—not in law and certainly not in practice. Bodily integrity is not a principle that Indian criminal justice respects or upholds.

II

Informed Consent and Freedom from Coercion

3

THE SHAME OF MEDICAL RESEARCH

UNTIL THE 1990S American medical researchers performed most of their experiments on other Americans—frequently choosing subjects who were poor and vulnerable.[1] Now, however, they are increasingly likely to conduct their investigations in third-world countries on subjects who are even poorer and more vulnerable. Part of the reason is AIDS—the first modern infectious disease to strike the developed and developing world simultaneously and to give both a large stake in finding a cure. Part of the reason, too, is the mounting financial and regulatory burdens of research in the rich nations, which cause investigators, both from universities and drug companies, to go to the poorer countries to test new treatments.

Whatever the reason, practice has overwhelmed ethics. The major international codes on human experimentation, including the principles proclaimed at Nuremberg in 1947 and the World Medical Association's Declaration of Helsinki in 1964, all say that the well-being of the subject always should take precedence over the needs of science

---

1. The mixed record of human experimentation in the US continues to be explored, with recent attention devoted to the government's secret radiation experiments during the cold war. See Chapter 4 of this book; Eileen Welsom, *The Plutonium Files* (Dial Press, 1999); and Jonathan D. Marino, *Undue Risk* (Freeman, 1999).

or the interests of society, and that doctors must obtain "the subject's freely informed consent." But neither these codes nor the Western groups concerned with medical ethics have had the developing countries in mind. Countries in which clinical trials are now conducted are often too poor to pay for the medicines that are successfully tested. And the people recruited for those trials very seldom get the kind of medical care the participants in trials in prosperous countries can expect. Whether Western principles covering the treatment of people who are the subjects of research can and should be applied in Africa and Asia has become a bitterly debated question. Indeed, the arguments that follow below sparked a number of acrimonious responses and even threats of academic retaliation. The original *New York Review of Books* article (November 30, 2000) was also translated and reprinted in several languages and became the cover story of one French weekly. Accordingly, the text is left unchanged and one letter that was published in *The New York Review of Books*, along with the response to it, is included. A postscript brings the story up-to-date.

The question was first posed by the research that followed the 1994 finding that is known by its grant number—076—in the Pediatric AIDS Clinical Trials Group, a consortium of university-based investigators funded by the National Institutes of Health (NIH). The purpose of the research, everyone agrees, was admirable: to learn how to prevent the transmission of HIV from HIV-positive pregnant women to their children. The dispute that arose concerned whether the research was conducted ethically.

In 076, American investigators proved conclusively, through clinical trials in the US, that giving AZT to HIV-positive pregnant women during their pregnancy and immediately before labor, and then to their newborn infants for six weeks, significantly reduced the rate of transmission of HIV. Without AZT, roughly one third of the women transmitted the virus to their newborn babies. With AZT, mothers passed on the virus only 8 percent of the time, for a total reduction of 66 percent. Clearly, AZT provided extensive protection against the spread of AIDS from mother to child.[2]

Even the 076 trial stirred some argument. AZT is a highly toxic drug, with many serious side effects, and investigators were administering it to pregnant women of whom only one third would have passed on the disease. Was it ethical to subject the fetuses of the other two thirds to a toxic drug, when, if left alone, they would not have suffered any adverse consequences?

This question had to be submitted to the institutional review boards (IRBs) at the researchers' home institutions. By federal regulations, all human experiments supported with federal funds must first be approved by an IRB, and practically every university, hospital, or company doing such research has established one. The regulations spell out how an IRB should be organized (for example, with no fewer than five members, with at least one not affiliated with the institution) and what standards it should enforce (research benefits must outweigh risks and investigators must give potential subjects enough information to ensure informed consent).

But the final decision on what is or is not ethical research is left to the individual IRBs. There is no regular review of their decisions, and, despite some requests to create one, there is no national IRB to supercede them. In the AZT research on pregnant women, all the IRBs took the position that since no one could identify in advance which newborn would be spared the disease and which would contract it, it was ethical to subject all of them to the risk of toxic effects.

Giving AZT to HIV-positive pregnant women and newborn infants immediately became the standard of care in American hospitals.

---

2. E. M. Connor et al., "Reduction of Maternal-Infant Transmission of Human Immunodeficiency Virus Type I with Zidovudine Treatment," *New England Journal of Medicine*, Vol. 337 (1994), pp. 1173–1180.

(Some doctors and public health officials even advocated compulsory HIV testing of pregnant women to ensure that their offspring were protected.) But this treatment stood little chance of being adopted in developing countries with mounting cases of AIDS. A six-month course of AZT costs about $800, far beyond the budgetary means of countries whose average annual expenditure per citizen for health care was below $25. Some American investigators, strongly suspecting that the virus was most likely to be passed during late pregnancy or childbirth, suggested that a short course of AZT might be almost as protective as the long course. Were this true, the cost of treatment would be markedly reduced and the benefits almost as great.

The clinical trials to test the efficacy of a short course of AZT required two groups, or arms, as they are called. The active arm would receive the short course. But what would the second arm, the control group, receive? Should it get the full course of AZT that American women were receiving, or should it get a placebo? Almost all the researchers in the field—most of them in southern Africa and Thailand—decided to give the control groups a placebo. In February 1998, the result of the first trial was announced: the short course of AZT was effective, not to the degree of the full course but substantially more effective than the placebo. A small amount of AZT (at a cost of $50, as against $800 for the long course) reduced transmission by 40 to 50 percent, which was excellent news for countries like Thailand, which was able to afford the treatment. It was good news to African countries, which would have more difficulty paying for it but could hope to supplement their medical budgets with humanitarian aid.

But the positive findings did nothing to reduce the intensity of the debate over whether the control groups should have received some medical treatment. The basic issue was one of the ethical obligations to a control group facing deadly disease when an effective therapy existed. Since the efficacy of AZT against mother-to-infant transmission was fully established, why not give the control groups the long course of AZT and use this as the base against which to measure outcomes for the short course?

This was precisely the position adopted by Marcia Angell in a now famous *New England Journal of Medicine* editorial.[3] Angell cited the Declaration of Helsinki provision that control groups should always receive the "best proven diagnostic and therapeutic method," which in this case meant the long course of AZT. When researchers in southern Africa and Thailand gave control groups a placebo, Angell wrote, they violated the Helsinki standards and demonstrated "a callous disregard of their welfare." She then went on to compare the research to the Tuskegee study, the most notorious American research scandal, in which, from the 1930s through the 1960s, the US Public Health Service had purposely withheld known effective treatments from black men suffering from syphilis. Angell charged that investigators were now withholding effective treatments from black women and children in Africa suffering from AIDS. "It seems," concluded Angell, "as if we have not come very far from Tuskegee after all. Those of us in the research community need to redouble our commitment to the highest ethical standards, no matter where the research is conducted."

Her position was supported by Sidney Wolfe and Peter Lurie, the physicians who head the Health Research Group of Public Citizen, the organization founded by Ralph Nader.[4] They calculated that as of 1997, sixteen research projects were investigating the effectiveness of short-course AZT, using as subjects some 17,000 pregnant women in developing countries. In fifteen of the sixteen projects, nine of which were funded by the NIH or the Centers for Disease Control (CDC), the

---

3. Marcia Angell, "The Ethics of Clinical Research in the Third World," *New England Journal of Medicine*, Vol. 337 (1997), pp. 847–849.

4. Peter Lurie and Sidney Wolfe, "Unethical Trials of Interventions to Reduce Perinatal Transmission of the Human Immunodeficiency Virus in Developing Countries," *New England Journal of Medicine*, Vol. 337 (1997), pp. 853–856.

control groups did not receive AZT. (The one exception was a Harvard School of Public Health project in Thailand.)

Wolfe and Lurie could find no justification for allowing investigators to adopt lower standards abroad than they used in the US. "Researchers working in developing countries," they wrote, "have an ethical responsibility to provide treatment that conforms to the standard of care in the sponsoring countries, when possible." They conceded that if achieving that standard required exorbitant expenses, like building an intensive care unit, the requirement could be waived. But if the test involved a drug that the manufacturer could, and sometimes did, provide free of charge, then a different standard was truly a double standard, and this, they concluded, "creates an incentive to use as research subjects those with the least access to health care."

The position of Angell, Wolfe, and Lurie provoked responses every bit as vigorous and uncompromising. The head of the NIH, Harold Varmus, and the head of the CDC, David Satcher, defended 076, as did Michael Merson, executive director of the WHO Global Program on AIDS.[5] The long course of AZT, they said, was not only very expensive but required frequent medical monitoring that was beyond the capacity of developing countries. So giving AZT could in fact be compared to building an intensive care unit. They also argued that it might not be safe to use AZT in a population that was seriously undernourished and suffering from anemia, and that placebo trials were also quicker than others in getting an answer.

Since critics contested each of these points, defenders of the post-076 trials went on to insist that research ethics in developing countries should not be dictated by the United States. Local ethics committees, they claimed, were competent to review research projects, and since

---

5. Harold Varmus and David Satcher, "Ethical Complexities of Conducting Research in Developing Countries," *New England Journal of Medicine*, Vol. 337 (1997), pp. 1003–1005; and Vol. 338 (1998), pp. 836–844.

Africans and Asians had approved these trials, outsiders should not second-guess them. Varmus and Satcher quoted from a letter written by the chairman of the Uganda Cancer Institute research committee: "These are Ugandan studies conducted by Ugandan investigators on Ugandans.... It is not NIH conducting the studies in Uganda but Ugandans conducting their study on their people for the good of their people."

One last contention was too political to be voiced openly but was often hinted at privately. No country wanted to spend significant amounts of money on second-class treatment. If a short course of AZT was openly compared to a long course, health officials would have to ask political leaders to fund a program that was less effective than the American one. But if results from the short course were compared to those from a placebo, they would be able to request funding to reduce by half the number of newborn babies infected by HIV.

Just how irreconcilable the differences between the two camps are becomes apparent in the provisions of the 1993 International Ethical Guidelines for Biomedical Research Involving Human Subjects. Drafted by the Council for International Organizations of Medical Sciences and the WHO, the document attempts to formulate research ethics in developing countries with particular attention to combating AIDS. However, the document is ambivalent about the issues raised by the post-076 trials. First, it declares, "investigators must respect the ethical standards of their own countries." They "risk harming their reputation by pursuing work that host countries find acceptable but their own countries find offensive." But it then adds that investigators must respect "the cultural expectations of the societies in which research is undertaken" and ought not to "transgress the cultural values of the host country by uncritically conforming to the expectations of their own." So should researchers conduct such placebo trials? The document does not say.

* * *

59

More and more instances of AIDS research that follows the post-076 model are coming to light, and their defenders are attempting to amend the Helsinki Declaration so that it will agree with their views. At the same time, the efforts to develop an AIDS vaccine are raising new and troubling questions about ethics in research. And quite apart from AIDS, the sheer amount of research in developing countries both by academic and drug company investigators is expanding enormously.

AIDS investigations in developing countries often withhold effective treatments from research subjects. It is true that AZT or antiviral drugs are expensive and difficult to administer under conditions of poverty; but probably as crucial is the fact that providing treatment fatally undermines the research. For example, under an NIH grant, investigators from the University of Washington and the University of Nairobi examined genital shedding of HIV-1 DNA and RNA during pregnancy, in order to analyze HIV transmission from mothers to their unborn children.[6] (This research program, or "protocol," and the others discussed below were obtained through the Freedom of Information Act.) Using HIV-positive women as research subjects, investigators took swabs of mucus from around the cervix and genital tract and also drew a blood sample during and after their pregnancy. The consent form told prospective participants:

> We...want to know more about the virus in the birth canal. We want to know whether every infected woman has the virus in her birth canal, or whether only some women have the virus here. We want to know whether there are reasons why some women might have the virus in the birth canal.

The researchers took their swabs at the twenty-fourth, thirty-second,

---

6. "Genital Shedding and Intrapartum Transmission of HIV-1," NIH grant K08 HD01160, Progress Report Summary, August 1, 1997, through July 31, 1998.

and thirty-sixth weeks of pregnancy and then again two weeks and six months after delivery. If they discovered evidence of a sexually transmitted disease other than AIDS, they treated it. But they did not treat HIV, and they did not themselves provide the pregnant women with the AZT that could prevent transmission to their offspring. Although they acknowledged the efficacy of short-course AZT, their progress report to NIH noted:

> It remains essential to understand the mechanism of vertical [mother to infant] HIV-1 transmission in order to design feasible intervention strategies to decrease transmission.

If they had administered AZT, they would have been unable to conduct their study.

Under another protocol, researchers from Johns Hopkins in collaboration with Mulago Hospital and Makerere University in Kampala, Uganda, investigated the efficacy of an intensified version of gamma globulin (HIV-IG) in preventing HIV transmission from mothers to infants. They gave three groups of HIV-infected mothers different doses of the HIV-IG, but none of them received AZT. "The expense of AZT, compliance, and toxicity considerations," the researchers claimed, "make widespread use of this approach in developing countries impractical."[7] But rather than try to learn whether Ugandan pregnant women might comply with the demanding AZT regimen and whether it was actually more toxic for them than for Americans, they experimented with their new agent. The research could not have been conducted in the US because it withheld from the women a drug of known efficacy. By adopting a different set of rules, it could be conducted in Uganda.

---

7. "HIV-IG for Prevention of Vertical Transmission," NIH grant R01 AI34235-06, Progress Report Summary, February 1, 1997, through January 30, 1998, p. 27.

In the fall of 1997, several months before the efficacy of short-course AZT was demonstrated, a team from the Walter Reed Army Institute of Research, Johns Hopkins, and Lampang Hospital in northern Thailand, with NIH funding, investigated transmission of HIV from mothers to infants by collecting blood and vaginal fluids from pregnant women. The consent form alerted the subjects to the possibility of taking AZT:

> A drug, called AZT, has been proven effective in reducing the risk of HIV transmission from infected mothers to their babies in studies performed in the United States and Europe. At present, it is unknown whether AZT would reduce risk of HIV transmission from infected mothers to their babies in Thailand.

The Thai Ministry of Public Health, the form explained, was planning such studies and the subjects were given the name of a doctor to contact for information. The consent form said: "We would encourage you to consider joining this AZT study."

At least two problems arise with this approach. First, the team did not itself offer to provide the subjects with AZT; those who wanted it would have to enroll in the Thai trials. The IRB in the US Surgeon General's office reviewed the project and asked whether this arrangement satisfied its own regulation that "any study must meet the same standards of ethics and safety that apply to research conducted within the US involving US citizens." The IRB decided that it did, on the grounds that "ethical objections are alleviated by unequivocal consent form endorsement of the use of perinatal AZT." It did not acknowledge that IRBs would not have approved a project in the United States in which researchers endorsed but failed to provide an effective treatment to their subjects.

Why did the researchers in Thailand not give women AZT? Because the project was enrolling pregnant women who, lacking the drug, were transmitting the disease to their children—which was precisely what the investigators needed to have happen in order to do their study. As they told the NIH reviewers of their project, "The advent of AZT use was a concern of the [NIH] study section . . . [because] our analysis plan was based on identifying approximately 25–30 transmissions in the population." But the concern, the investigators declared, was unnecessary. "We will have at least 100 deliveries without exposure to AZT in any form yielding about 20 transmissions." Only because the virus continued to be passed on was the study workable.[8]

Another NIH-supported project from the University of Washington explored the genital transmission of HIV. The subjects were four hundred HIV-positive prostitutes in Mombasa, Kenya, none of whom received AZT or antiviral therapy. Three hundred of the group who had other sexually transmitted diseases, in addition to AIDS, were treated for those diseases in order to learn how treatment affects the transmission of HIV. (The question being posed is whether antibiotics administered for syphilis reduce the rate of HIV transmission.) Another sixty women received oral contraceptives or injectable progesterone to learn whether methods of contraception affect the rate of HIV transmission. Finally, another ten women were examined daily for one month to learn if the quantity of cervical and vaginal HIV changes during the menstrual cycle. The investigators believed these studies would help to create new ways to prevent sexual transmission of HIV. Such a study could not be conducted in the United States, because it withholds a known effective treatment.

In Rwanda and Zambia, University of Alabama investigators are enrolling couples (rather than prostitutes) for their studies of HIV

---

8. Department of the Army, Office of the Surgeon General, Memorandum for Director, Walter Reed Army Institute of Research, "Addendum to . . . 'Evaluation of HIV-1 Viral Burden . . . ,'" November 12, 1997, p. 30, with the "Informed Consent" revised September 10, 1997; NIH grant HD34343-03, Progress Report Summary, p. 20.

transmission. They follow the medical history of couples in which one partner is HIV-positive and the other HIV-negative—about 20 percent of all couples tested—to learn when, and under what conditions, the negative partner turns positive. These studies, they say, are "natural history studies," that is, they merely observe people. Since prescriptions for antiviral therapy are rare in both countries, the researchers are ostensibly following the "natural," that is, untreated, history of the disease. They do, they say, dispense "commonly available medications for infectious diseases" to the subjects, although not to local people generally; and while they provide "general health education on ways to avoid AIDS," they do not distribute contraceptives. The genocide in Rwanda crippled research there. ("Half of our pre-genocide staff," the team reported, "are known dead or remain missing and less than half of our study subjects have returned to Kigali.") But work goes forward in Zambia. Investigators were able to distinguish between subjects who were "rapid progressors" to death and those who were "long term survivors." They anticipate that understanding the viral and epidemiological differences between the two groups will produce effective public health and treatment strategies. Again the research depends on withholding effective treatment from subjects and not supplying contraceptives.[9]

One AIDS research project in Uganda recently made headlines mostly because its findings were published in the *New England Journal of Medicine* and were commented upon, negatively but now more cautiously, by Marcia Angell.[10] A team led by Thomas Quinn from Johns Hopkins, collaborating with investigators from the NIH,

---

9. "Heterosexual Transmission and Natural History of HIV Infection in Rwanda/Zambia," NIH grant Ro1 AI40951-04, Progress Report Summary, October 1995, p. 25.

10. T. C. Quinn et al., "Viral Load and Heterosexual Transmission of Human Immunodeficiency Virus Type I," *New England Journal of Medicine*, Vol. 342 (2000), pp. 921–929, 967–969; and Vol. 343 (2000), pp. 361–363.

Columbia University, and Makerere University, Kampala, studied 15,000 persons in rural Uganda to see whether prophylactic use of antibiotics prevented the spread of sexually transmitted diseases. It turned out, two and a half years later, that the strategy did not work; but trying to salvage something from the research, which had included testing the subjects every ten months for HIV disease, the investigators went back to their records and, using family names and addresses, linked husband to wife in order to see what they could discover about HIV transmission. They identified 415 couples in which, when the project started, one partner had been HIV-positive and the other had not. Of the HIV-negative subjects, ninety had became positive during the study. The critical causal factor was the "viral load," that is, the degree of infection that the HIV-positive person was carrying. Higher loads led to higher rates of HIV transmission. It was this finding that the researchers submitted for publication in the *New England Journal of Medicine*.

Since the policy of the *New England Journal of Medicine* is not to publish the results of unethical research, and since this particular protocol, like other post-076 ones, withheld effective treatment, Angell felt it necessary to explain why the report on it was accepted. She scrupulously identified all the considerations that would prevent such research from being done in the US, including, in most states, the need to inform the uninfected spouse that the partner was HIV-positive and to treat HIV disease when discovered. She did not believe that the later identification of the couples was a mitigating circumstance. Nor did she accept as a mitigating circumstance the fact that, according to the researchers, official Ugandan policy advises against partner notification. Faced with such a policy, she said, the researchers should have reconsidered the ethics of doing research in Uganda. In light of the frequent HIV testing, "seronegative partners of seropositive persons could easily have been identified and informed of their special risk." Angell also noted that the study's principal finding—that high viral loads are predictive of transmission—would not benefit Uganda since it could not afford the drug treatments that would reduce the viral load. Why then did she publish the study? Two (unnamed) experts on ethics whom she consulted were divided on the question, she wrote, and she wanted to "focus attention on the vexing ethical issues." Angell still believed that "our ethical standards should not depend on where the research is performed." But this time, instead of invoking the precedent of the Tuskegee scandal, she concluded that "all these questions are debatable, and that there may be few answers that apply to every situation."

In an effort to free researchers from the constraints of existing ethical codes, a number of investigators and bioethicists, led by Robert Levine, a Yale physician, have proposed to the WMA several fundamental revisions to the Declaration of Helsinki.[11] The code currently reads: "In any medical study, every patient—including those of a control group, if any—should be assured of the best proven diagnostic and therapeutic method." Their amended version would read: "...should be assured that he or she will not be denied access to the best proven diagnostic, prophylactic or therapeutic method that *would otherwise be available to him or her*" (italics added). The Helsinki Declaration allows the use of placebos only "in studies where no proven diagnostic or therapeutic method exists." The Levine proposal states: "When

---

11. A disclosure may be in order. Robert Levine and David Rothman were opposing expert witnesses in a recent case brought against Vanderbilt University for research it conducted between 1945 and 1947 (see Chapter 4 of this book). In that study, pregnant women were fed radioactive iron (to study iron absorption), and told that they were receiving a "vitamin cocktail." Levine argued that such practices were in keeping with the ethical norms at the time. David insisted that such deception violated already recognized ethical principles governing human experimentation, and that the Nuremberg Code (issued a few months after the protocol ended) incorporated longstanding principles and did not invent them. Vanderbilt settled the case for $10 million and issued an apology, read in court, to the plaintiffs.

the outcome measures are neither death nor disability, placebo or other no-treatment controls may be justified on the basis of their efficiency."

The two changes substantially reduce investigators' responsibilities. Under the Helsinki principles, they must supply their research subjects with the best therapies that have been developed; in the future, they would need only not interfere with subjects' receiving therapies. Subjects would no longer be "assured" of receiving the best proven therapy; instead, they would "not be denied access" to them. Moreover, the revision would allow investigators to provide subjects, including control groups, only with those therapies that were available to them in their own country; in effect, researchers would not be obligated to provide first-world treatments in the third world. Finally, the revision opens the door more widely to placebo trials. Placebos may be used even when effective treatments are locally available if the injuries that would follow from not giving such treatments fall short of death or disability. In effect, the proposed changes to Helsinki would render ethical all the protocols described here.

Modifying the Helsinki standards would immediately affect the design of AIDS vaccine trials, which raise in particularly distressing fashion the question of what is owed human subjects in developing countries. An AIDS vaccine is truly the best hope for stopping the ravages of the disease worldwide but nowhere more dramatically than in developing countries. Vaccines, it is true, are not easy to deliver in poor countries; ways have to be found to maintain the "cold chain," that is, to store the vaccines at an appropriately cool temperature, and to reach isolated populations. But the successes of smallpox and polio vaccines indicate that these difficulties can be surmounted. The very potential of an AIDS vaccine to save thousands of lives makes the ethics of testing it more complex. The NIH and several drug companies have begun testing HIV vaccines not only in the United States but in Thailand, and plans are under way to conduct vaccine trials in China, India, South Africa, Haiti, Peru, and Trinidad.

The first difficulty is that testing the vaccine requires using subjects who can be expected to be exposed to AIDS; otherwise no useful findings on its efficacy will be forthcoming. Of necessity, then, subjects will be drawn from vulnerable populations, including drug users, commercial sex workers, and sexually active, risk-prone gay men, all of whom may be easily coerced into joining the research. How to guard against such coercion is by no means obvious. Second, both American and Helsinki standards would require that subjects in such a trial initially receive educational counseling, clean needles, condoms, and perhaps even drug abuse treatment and vocational counseling. Thus, research ethics undercut research efficacy: if every subject heeded the advice and took the protective measures, the efficacy of the vaccine tests would be seriously impaired. Third, were subjects later to contract AIDS either as a result of a faulty vaccine or because of their own failure to take necessary precautions, a strong case could be made for their being given, at researchers' expense, AZT or the latest antiretroviral drugs. Judging by their past performance, researchers are not likely to expend the thousands of dollars necessary to meet this commitment.

By contrast, adopting local, not international standards would make the trials cheaper (because no treatment would have to be provided) and increase their efficacy (because by not supplying clean needles or condoms, subjects would be more frequently exposed to HIV). So, too, if subjects who contracted AIDS were not given AZT or antiretrovirals, researchers would learn more about other properties of the vaccine, including whether it reduced the severity of the disease or the infectiousness of the virus.

With these advantages in mind, Barry Bloom, chair of the UNAIDS Vaccine Advisory Committee, recently observed: "Determination of the protective efficacy of HIV vaccine candidates may only be possible in trials in developing countries where the resources are not available to provide antiretroviral drugs."[12] Although aware of the ethical dilemmas of having science take advantage of a country's poverty, he and many colleagues say they cannot put aside the benefits of the knowledge to be gained. "If the best proven therapeutic standard of the industrialized countries were literally applied without qualification," Bloom argues, "could there ever be efficacy trials of AIDS vaccines or of many other interventions?" His conclusion is guarded but his preference clear: the Helsinki standards "require clarification and perhaps modification."

The attractions of conducting research in developing countries are not limited to AIDS or to academic investigators. Over the past ten years, American drug companies have been reducing their reliance upon universities to do their research, turning instead to for-profit contract-research organizations (CROs). (In 1991, according to one analysis, 80 percent of drug industry funding for clinical trials went to academic medical centers; by 1998, the figure had dropped by half.[13]) The CROs locate the research sites, recruit patients, and in some cases even draw up the study design and perform the analysis. And increasingly the sites and patients they choose are abroad, particularly in developing countries.

In London in February 2000, a two-day meeting, sponsored by a number of major pharmaceutical companies and addressed by CRO representatives, was devoted to "Unleashing the Untapped Potential of Clinical Trials in Southeast Asia," including China, South Korea, and Malaysia. The program announcement said: "Per patient trial costs are up to 25 percent lower than in the US & Europe. Lower per

---

12. Barry R. Bloom, "The Highest Attainable Standard: Ethical Issues in AIDS Vaccines," *Science*, Vol. 279 (1998), pp. 186–188.

13. Thomas Bodenheimer, "Uneasy Alliance—Clinical Investigators and the Pharmaceutical Industry," *New England Journal of Medicine*, Vol. 342 (2000), p. 1540.

patient trial costs is just one of the benefits available to you by under-taking clinical trials in Southeast Asia." It also explained that the changing "disease profile" of Southeast Asians made them more like Americans and Europeans. For example, cardiovascular disorders, from which drug companies make huge profits, are fast replacing infectious diseases as the leading cause of death in these countries. Asians were also better subjects for clinical trials because they were "treatment naive," that is, previously unexposed to other medical interventions. Not explicitly stated but well known to all researchers is the additional fact that most Southeast Asian countries do not have effective review boards, or, for that matter, highly inquisitive and demanding patients. In this way, global economics goes hand in hand with global medicine.[14]

The debates over the ethics of placebo trials spill over into the ques-tion of consent. Those who support the standards of the developed countries insist that all those who take part in a trial, whatever their culture, must personally agree to join it. But those who say they are ready to adapt to local custom would tailor consent requirements accordingly. In cultures where, in many important matters, tribal chiefs give consent for their tribesmen or husbands give consent for their wives, the same may be done for research.

What, in any case, do research subjects in Thailand or Uganda understand about the research projects in which they take part? What do the Nairobi prostitutes make of research on viruses in the birth canal? Very few studies in the developing world address this issue, but some findings there and elsewhere are suggestive. In the United States, where consent has been better investigated, anywhere from 25 to 50 percent of patients and subjects do not understand what it is that they

---

14. Helen Epstein described how this process works in South Africa. See "The Mystery of AIDS in South Africa," *The New York Review of Books*, July 20, 2000.

have agreed to. Among two hundred patients being treated at the University of Pennsylvania Cancer Center, 40 percent did not know the purpose or nature of the procedure they had undergone and 45 percent could not give even one major risk or cite a possible complication resulting from it. Such findings may possibly be explained by the age or education of the patients, poor communication by physicians, or blind trust by patients. But whatever the reason, consent is hardly informed.

The same must be true in developing countries. No one ought to justify placebo-based protocols simply because Ugandan or Thai subjects consented to join them. Not only would these subjects face all of the difficulties in getting information that their Western counterparts do, but they may well be encountering alien concepts. Take the idea of randomization. Subjects are informed (by doctors or white-coated assistants) that a toss of a coin will determine whether they receive treatment or placebo. The proposition is not self-evident, requiring as it does an understanding of rules of chance and an appreciation of the unusual fact that a doctor may not be giving treatment. Americans are often confused about this; when Johns Hopkins researchers questioned American drug users being recruited for a randomized HIV vaccine trial, 26 percent did not understand that some subjects would be receiving vaccine and others placebo. An investigator in Bangkok recently explained to me that there is no Thai word for placebo. The best the team could come up with is a term most accurately translated as "mimic." Accordingly, subjects in some of the Thai post-076 trials were told that they would either get medication or a substance that mimicked medication. Whether the term was understood as a stand-in for medicine or as a nonmedicine is anybody's guess.

Finally, in some developing countries "consent" may be deceptive. In 1998 a team of South African doctors and public health workers questioned subjects who had enrolled in an HIV-transmission study about their knowledge of the disease. It turned out that they had an accurate understanding of HIV transmission. But in an unexpected finding, they also made it clear that they had had no choice about enrolling; 84 percent said they felt they had been compelled to participate. Just why they felt this wasn't clear, but they were evidently under pressure of some kind. A follow-up question asked whether the hospital would permit them to quit the study, and 98 percent said no. So much for the voluntary nature of informed consent.

The immediate effort to relax international standards may not succeed. The WMA debated revisions to the Helsinki Declaration at its 1999 annual meeting in Tel Aviv and the participants, without exception, said that the proposed changes violated the fundamental ethics of research on human beings. At the WMA's October 2000 meeting held in Edinburgh, delegates resolved that any new treatment had to be tested against "the best current prophylactic, diagnostic, and therapeutic methods," thereby maintaining a commitment to a universal standard for research. And some organizations in the US are trying to strengthen the ability of developing countries to review research protocols. The Fogarty International Center of the NIH, for example, has begun a program that will provide representatives from developing countries with training in ethics, particularly American research ethics. Such training will not guarantee that local ethics committees will be more concerned with protecting fellow citizens than with cooperating with well-financed foreign investigators. But it might give them a clearer sense of ethical issues.

Nevertheless, the larger debate is unresolved. Whatever the moral force of the WMA, it has no power of enforcement, and a number of other organizations are putting forth guidelines that are far more equivocal. The UNAIDS Guidance Document, "Ethical Considerations in HIV Preventive Vaccine Research," released in February 2000, recommends that community representatives be included in the research approval process and that subjects be given counseling on reducing risks. But the document refuses to take a stand on the central questions. It distinguishes between ideal treatment ("the best proven therapy") and the minimum treatment (access to "the highest level of care attainable in the host country") but leaves it to the host country, the sponsor of the research, and the local community to work out the level of treatment. In so doing, it makes both ideal and minimum standards ethically acceptable. It also assumes, incorrectly, that the three constituents are equal in power and offers no suggestions about resolving conflicts among them.

With similar equivocation, a 1998 ad hoc meeting of selected investigators (including several whose protocols are discussed here) and some bioethicists issued a consensus statement, published in *The Lancet*, called "Science, Ethics, and the Future of Research into Maternal Infant Transmission of HIV." Its position was that "study participants should be assured the highest standard of care practically attainable in the country in which the trial is carried out." This standard would presumably be higher than the "available" level of care but below that of the "best proven therapy." But how is one to know what is or is not "attainable" in a country short of trying? And if a standard of care is attainable by importing resources or technology, does that matter? The efforts to whittle away at the Helsinki Declaration demonstrate the value of its clear and unambiguous standard.

After exhausting other arguments, proponents eager to modify the Helsinki Declaration insist, often passionately, that the tidal wave of AIDS sweeping the world, particularly in southern Africa, is so dreadful that researchers must be given a relatively free hand in order to find useful treatments. But the proposition has several weaknesses. As soon as research protections are weakened, profit-seeking companies will take advantage of them, not to cure AIDS but to increase their returns.

Even more important, to date the results of placebo-based AIDS trials have not brought medical benefits to Africa. Short-course AZT was supposed to be helpful, but it is infrequently used. (I am told by one investigator that in Lusaka, Zambia, some 2,000 pregnant women in research studies are the only ones receiving it, this in a city where more than 30,000 women give birth each year.) At the moment, a new drug called nevirapine is being hailed as the solution to maternal–infant transmission of HIV, mostly because it is very cheap and, to be effective, needs only be given at the onset of labor. But whether it will actually be used in developing countries is unclear. South Africa, for reasons that no one can understand, has already rejected it. And it is worth noting that when nevirapine itself was tested, the control group was given AZT not in its proven short-course regimen, but only from the onset of labor through delivery. The investigators claimed that the short course was too complicated to be administered in a developing country.[15]

There are strong practical as well as principled reasons for Americans to follow American ethical standards when they do research abroad. IRBs have too little familiarity with developing countries to set different standards. They are ill equipped to differentiate among the values and customs of Thailand, China, Uganda, or Zambia. They cannot possibly know whether the word "placebo" has been accurately translated. Moreover, making human rights relative to social and economic conditions in distant countries could come back to haunt us. Appalachia is not Westchester County, and the mortality statistics in Harlem are worse than those in Bangladesh. Will American researchers be allowed to provide less treatment in our own impoverished regions than in prosperous ones? The question is not idle, for this is the position that the US Public Health Service adopted in conducting and rationalizing the Tuskegee research.

As Aryeh Neier, former head of the ACLU, has pointed out, American courts often must balance local values against national standards. When the stakes are not life-threatening, the courts have been respectful

---

15. The ongoing controversy in South Africa over the use of nevirapine to prevent mother-to-child transmission of HIV is discussed in greater detail in Chapter 6.

of local values, most notably in education. (The Amish get to educate their children by their own criteria, not those of the majority.) But in a matter of life or death, courts enforce national values. (A Jehovah's Witness parent may not decide for his child that death is preferable to receiving a transfusion.) A good case can be made that AIDS research in developing countries should follow this same principle.

Finally, abject poverty is harsh enough without people having to bear the additional burdens of serving as research subjects. When we take account of the misery and stunted hopes of people in Uganda, it is not enough for investigators to say that their research left them no worse off. That Ugandans did not have access to AZT before the research, during the research, or after the research does not resolve the ethical issue. As compensation to their subjects for enrolling in the research, investigators who come to Uganda should be required to leave their subjects better off. And the Ugandans should receive the benefits of treatment now, not in some distant future when pharmaceutical companies may, or may not, reduce the price of their drugs or vaccines so that citizens in poor countries can afford them. Do unto others as we do unto ourselves—a principle for researchers everywhere.

On March 8, 2001, the following exchange appeared in *The New York Review of Books*:

To the Editors:

Those in the scientific community who have sought to contribute to the struggle against AIDS and to reconcile the demands of the global AIDS problem with respect for the current ethical guidelines for biomedical research look to the broader scholarly community for understanding and guidance. It is disappointing, therefore, that there is so little insight or useful guidance forthcoming from historian David Rothman, who, in a provocatively entitled essay, "The Shame of Medical Research," chose, rather, to impugn the motives of the AIDS research community. In his sweeping indictment of AIDS research, Professor Rothman, quoting highly selectively from institutional review filings and scientific papers, alleges that what motivates scientists to study AIDS in developing countries in Africa and elsewhere is really the ability to study scientific questions that cannot easily be studied in the US, where most HIV/AIDS-infected individuals have access to highly active antiretroviral therapy. It would have been generous—and surely pertinent—had he indicated that there is another, much more compelling reason—namely, that 95 percent of all HIV/AIDS victims live—and die—in developing countries.

HIV/AIDS is not, as Professor Rothman implies, a convenient vehicle for satisfying scientific curiosity. AIDS is the greatest epidemic in the history of humankind. It will be more devastating than the Black Death of 1346 or influenza of 1919. At present, we have no cure, no vaccine. The drugs that control the disease in the US are so expensive that they are unavailable to the overwhelming majority of the world's population that live in developing countries. This is the compelling reality that motivates the scientific community to carry out research on arguably the most challenging infectious disease problem biomedical science has ever faced.

What is an ethical study in a population of a developing country that is ravaged by an invariably fatal disease? The Declaration of Helsinki on the ethics of research involving human subjects was formulated in 1964 with only an industrialized world in mind. Both Helsinki and the CIOMS (Council of International Organizations of Medical Sciences and WHO) Guidelines, regarded by most as the standard ethical guidelines for research on human subjects, are silent on the technical or financial ability of poor developing countries to fulfill them. For example, the original guidelines require that individuals in a clinical study be entitled to "the best proven therapeutic and diagnostic method." In the case of the 076 protocol for AZT-prevention of maternal–child transmission of HIV, which stimulated public debate here and elsewhere, most developing countries could neither implement the best proven treatment—which included treatment of the mother starting at eleven to twelve weeks before birth (it is rare in many countries that women appear at medical clinics that early in pregnancy), with five doses a day of AZT, an intravenous injection of AZT during labor (not something readily done in villages in Africa), and six weeks' treatment of the newborn—nor afford the $800 cost of the drug. That led to proposed clinical trials seeking to develop a more practical and affordable regimen that could be used to save lives. Some in the medical establishment believed that 076 was "the best proven therapeutic method" and that any modification to reduce cost and simplify technology to make it more applicable was unethical. Mercifully, trials with modified regimens did go on, and a far simpler and less expensive regimen than 076, using nevirapine, was found. Professor Rothman sees that process as a slippery slope and recommends that we hold to the original guideline for ethical research —"the best proven therapeutic method." Does he recommend this even if it cannot be properly administered? And even if the drugs are not affordable or available in the developing country?

Leaving aside the sometimes emotional arguments made in the context of AIDS research, one might ask how relevant the current guidelines would be for trials testing the effectiveness of aspirin in a developing country, such as India, for prevention of death from heart attacks and strokes. Aspirin is a cheap drug, highly effective in industrialized countries at preventing about 30 percent of deaths from heart attacks, and 50 percent of deaths from strokes, yet it has not been appropriately tested or widely used in developing countries. Concerns about efficacy and adverse effects that might occur in Asian populations suggest that such trials would be justified. What would be the standard of care or "the best proven therapeutic method" for anyone in a large aspirin trial who suffered a heart attack? In the West it would be angioplasty or coronary artery bypass graft surgery. Would Professor Rothman insist that unless everyone in the populations could be assured access to those interventions, such a trial not be conducted? Would he make the judgment that a trial seeking to reduce death from heart attacks and strokes that failed to apply those treatments was unethical? Would it be better were the trials seeking understanding of how to intervene in AIDS in Africa not done in any country that does not provide highly active antiretroviral therapy?

The preamble of the WHO Constitution states, "The highest attainable standard of health is a fundamental human right, without distinction of race, religion, political belief, economic or social conditions." Article 12 of the International Covenant of Economic, Social and Cultural Rights recognizes "the right of everyone to the enjoyment of the highest attainable standard of physical and mental health." Clearly reference to the highest attainable standard has had meaning beyond the minimum in the past. With these precedents in mind, UNAIDS suggested two-level guidance: "in the ideal, the best proven diagnostic and therapeutic method." Where that is not possible, it recommends "the highest level of care attainable in the host country." This is dismissed by Professor Rothman as "the minimum treatment." He asks, "But how is one to know what is or is not 'attainable' in a country short of trying? And if a standard of care is attainable by importing resources or technology, does that matter?" Does he really not know whether provision of drugs costing $15,000 per person per year in a country with $6 per capita health spending is attainable or sustainable? It is astonishing that he twice refers to the "highest attainable standard" put forward by UNAIDS, after open meetings around the world with scholars and activists from developing and industrialized countries, as a "minimum," when it is obvious that "minimum" means accepting current practice. One doesn't have to be an academic to understand the difference, and that the highest standard attainable in the country must be better than current practice, unless it is, in fact, "the best proven therapeutic method." Failure to apply a standard higher than the current practice would be subject to challenge. Professor Rothman insists that "the efforts to whittle away at the Helsinki Declaration demonstrate the value of its clear and unambiguous standard." How ethical is this position if it means ceasing to do research for a preventive or treatment in developing countries? Why does Professor Rothman not consider the ethical issues in failing to carry out research? What is the real-world implication of his concluding statement "Do unto others as we do unto ourselves"? Who would pay and who would provide these therapies?

The medical research community has been searching for principles that would enable research to be conducted ethically to meet the needs of developing countries—not only AIDS research, but all clinical research. The fact that there are ongoing revisions of the Helsinki and CIOMS guidelines, and many new ethical guidelines being proposed around the world, suggests that these are hard questions upon which people of good will may differ. I would submit that, having engaged openly in debate of these complex ethical and equity issues, it is not the medical research community that should be ashamed.

Barry R. Bloom

Dean, Harvard School of Public Health
Boston, Massachusetts

David Rothman replies:

Neither Dr. Bloom nor anyone else who has written to *The New York Review* or to me disputes a single fact about the many research protocols that I described. There is no disagreement that these investigations could not be conducted in the United States. Dr. Bloom's charge that I believe the researchers are driven only by scientific curiosity is both false and serves as a straw man to divert attention from the crucial issues. I did not intend to impugn the motives of individual investigators; indeed, I assume they are driven by a desire to help cure AIDS.

My belief, however, is that in trying to achieve this obviously important end, they made immediate and long-term judgments about means that are open to question. Perhaps the investigators were convinced, as Dr. Bloom is, that third-world research should be conducted under different standards. But my argument is that one cannot rely on an analysis of motives when researchers decide that the best standard of care cannot be delivered and when the hypotheses they are testing depend on care not being delivered.

Should traditional research ethics be modified to combat this devastating epidemic? Not according to the World Medical Association. After a full discussion of AIDS in developing countries, it affirmed at its November 1999 meeting the universal rights of human subjects. It insisted that, in all countries, when new treatments are tested, "the best current prophylactic, diagnostic, and therapeutic methods" should be given to the control groups. Science should not take advantage of social misery to advance knowledge, no matter how vital that knowledge might be.

Dr. Bloom rejects this principle, taking issue with a human rights–based approach to medical research. His claim is that if investigators cannot follow different rules in different countries, the fight against AIDS will be impaired and more deaths from the disease will follow. But why should so uncompromising a utilitarian standard be limited to the third world, or to AIDS? If the threat of a disease is dire, why not allow investigators more latitude wherever they are? Why not experiment more vigorously with dying patients or with people living in pockets of poverty in the United States? By the 1970s, Americans had rejected such an approach. Syphilis and hepatitis are terrible diseases. Nevertheless, we resolved that it was unethical for investigators to observe but not to treat black men with syphilis who lacked access to health care. We also decided that it was wrong to purposely infect with hepatitis the residents of a filthy and overcrowded institution for the mentally retarded because they would probably get it anyway.

Moreover, a human rights approach to research is not so impractical a standard for American researchers in third-world countries. However rudimentary the indigenous health care system, American investigators generally set up their own facilities in order to methodically administer new drugs to their subjects; if required, they might be able to obtain, from one or another source, the funds necessary to give people who serve as controls the same standard of treatment that they would get in the US. Indeed, one of Dr. Bloom's Harvard colleagues did just that in Thailand.

The question is not, as Dr. Bloom contends, whether AIDS research can be done in countries that do not provide all their citizens with antiretroviral therapy but rather what researchers are obliged to provide their subjects. Dr. Bloom consistently links the ethical standard for American researchers with the existing standard of care within a particular third-world country; so does the UNAIDS guideline. Indeed, his letter goes further than the guideline, arguing that the standard of care that is "attainable" must also be "sustainable." But research can be and should be held to a different standard, and for these very reasons I consider Dr. Bloom's position inadequate.

Are there limits on researchers' obligations? Yes. As I carefully noted, repeating the observations of Lurie and Wolfe, researchers are not obliged to build and operate an intensive care unit in a developing country. Hence, Dr. Bloom's hypothetical example about aspirin studies is irrelevant. Because investigators cannot do everything does not mean that they are exonerated from doing something.

Rather than invent imaginary situations, Dr. Bloom would have done better to have specifically addressed the ethics of the investigations that I described. On what grounds does he find it ethical for investigators not to give short-course AZT to the HIV-positive women they are observing so as to prevent transmission of the virus from mother to infant? Does Dr. Bloom believe that the surgeon general's institutional review board was correct in finding that investigators had satisfied ethical requirements when they endorsed the use of AZT but did not supply it to their HIV-positive and pregnant Thai subjects in order to prevent transmission?

I cited in my article a research project in Zambia that, while withholding effective treatment, followed the medical history of couples in which one partner had been HIV-positive and the other had not. How could Dr. Bloom distinguish such a research project from the so-called natural experiments of Tuskegee and Willowbrook? Would he, like the researchers, have withheld from Ugandan couples information on the HIV status of the partner, and if so, on what ethical grounds? Dr. Bloom celebrates, as most everyone does, the breakthrough in AIDS treatment made possible by the successful testing of nevirapine. (Even South Africa is now "considering" its use.) But he is silent on whether the nevirapine researchers were ethically justified in not giving the control group the AZT short-course regimen that was specifically designed for developing countries.

In the one specific case that he does discuss, Dr. Bloom misconstrues the debate over the research that established the efficacy of short-course AZT. The concern was not whether short-course AZT should be tested; there was sufficient evidence that it would work to justify the trial itself. No one that I know was against reducing cost and simplifying technology. What was at issue, as my article explained, was that the control group was given a placebo, not long-course AZT, and thus instead of receiving treatment by the best proven methods, got no treatment at all.

As for my article's title, editors, not authors, choose titles; but I accepted "The Shame of Medical Research." Why? Because, first, it linked ethics to the structure of medical research, not to individual researchers. As we came to understand in the 1960s and 1970s, the source of ethical dilemmas in human experimentation was not "bad" researchers but a system that was thoroughly utilitarian in its ethic.

Second, the title suggests that the situation in which some medical research takes place gives cause for shame. The gross disparities in life chances among rich and poor countries and the readiness to take advantage of these disparities are shameful and need to be brought to light. Justifying that readiness by the urgency of the war on AIDS is inadequate not only for reasons of principle but because no one can demonstrate that, in the third world, either the subjects of the research or their countrymen have benefited, or will necessarily benefit, from the research.

Some thirty years ago, the philosopher Hans Jonas persuasively argued that there is inevitably something ethically questionable about human experimentation, for it uses people as a means to an end (greater collective knowledge), not as ends in themselves. In the first world, the requirements of informed consent and equal access to benefits, although they may not be consistently observed, allow us to continue experiments with human beings. But when human experimentation is transported to the third world and even these requirements are absent, then shame seems an apt description.

Postscript: December 2005

The WMA has continued to debate the ethics of research in the third world, and although it has not amended the Declaration of Helsinki, it has added two notes of clarification. The first one reads:

> Extreme care must be taken in making use of a placebo-controlled trial and that in general this methodology should only be used in the absence of existing proven therapy. However, a placebo-controlled trial may be ethically acceptable, even if a proven therapy is available under the following circumstances:

> Where for compelling and scientifically sound methodological reasons its use is necessary to determine the efficacy or safety of a prophylactic, diagnostic, or therapeutic method; or... for a minor condition, and the patients will not be subject to any additional risk of serious or irreversible harm.

It is difficult to know whether these phrases aim to contradict or affirm the original formulation. The clause addressing "minor" conditions is not especially troubling; if a condition is truly minor, withholding known care for an experimental intervention does not put the subject at risk. But what constitutes "compelling" reasons for allowing placebo trials even when a known effective agent is available? Would cost be one? Would difficulty of delivery be another? Would increasing the speed with which findings might be made represent still another? Researchers could cite any one of these reasons to justify withholding effective treatments from control groups.

The second note is no less ambiguous. The original formulation of researchers' obligations to the citizens of a country in which the clinical trials are conducted reads: "At the conclusion of the study, every patient entered into the study should be assured of access to the best proven prophylactic, diagnostic and therapeutic methods identified by the study." The WMA has now added:

> The WMA hereby reaffirms its position that it is necessary during the study planning process to identify post-trial access by study participants to prophylactic, diagnostic and therapeutic procedures identified as beneficial in the study or access to other appropriate care. Post-trial access arrangements or other care must be described in the study protocol so the ethical review committee may consider such arrangements during its review.

The commitment that subjects be assured access to the new agents after the trial has been replaced with a commitment to information about arrangements before the trial. The provision for review by a local ethics committee does not provide substantial protection. These committees are typically dominated by country investigators who may be more interested in facilitating and joining in the research than in serving citizens.

This negative interpretation of the two new notes reflects what I learned from participating in a small meeting that the WMA convened prior to their issuance. Representatives of pharmaceutical companies and the NIH along with a few bioethicists complained bitterly about the duties imposed on researchers by the declaration. A few of us defended the original principles, but, in light of the results, with only limited success. Radical revision of the declaration was prevented, but not the conscious introduction of ambiguity.

The lack of clarity in the WMA revisions is found in other recent formulations of research ethics. The then head of the National Bioethics Advisory Committee and president of Princeton, Harold Shapiro, writing in the *New England Journal of Medicine* in 2001, seemingly accepted the principle that control groups should be given established and effective treatment, whether or not the treatment was already available in the country; he did allow delivering a "less effective" treatment, but only if the condition being studied was not "life threatening." Shapiro also added that such a waiver "would not apply to the treatment of life-threatening diseases such as HIV infection.... If our standard were adopted, many trials currently under way...might have to be stopped or redesigned."

To this point, Shapiro appeared to be supporting the principles of the original Declaration of Helsinki. However, he then went on to observe that the declaration "may be too rigid." It might impede research in diarrheal or upper respiratory diseases. Therefore, investigators should be allowed to depart from the principle "but only if it is required in order to address an urgent health problem in the host country." So we are again left in limbo: in the case of AIDS research, does his initial unwillingness to give a waiver prevail or, given the urgency of the AIDS epidemic, can the declaration principles be waived?

The NIH itself seems to accept the waiver position. The HIV Vaccine Trials Network that it has organized equivocates about the duties owed research participants. Its information sheet, "Questions and Answers: HVTN 040 Vaccine Trial," poses the following question: "What will happen to volunteers if they become HIV-infected from their behavior during the course of the trial?" The answer: "The participant will be referred to an appropriate doctor for care." Does "referred" mean that the care will not be paid for? And what is the standard for "an appropriate doctor," third world or first world?

So, too, the document addressing the 026 vaccine trial for Brazil, Haiti, and Trinidad and Tobago asks the question: "If in years to come the vaccines in the study are shown to be effective, will the countries that participated in the trials of these products have access to the vaccines at a reduced cost?" The answer: "This is an important issue. It is currently impossible to predict the cost of an effective vaccine.... A solution will need to be found."

In Britain, the prestigious Nuffield Council on Bioethics issued a report in 2005 entitled "The Ethics of Research Related to Healthcare in Developing Countries." Its position does not differ substantially from the others just discussed: "Wherever appropriate, participants in the control group should be offered a universal standard of care. Where it is inappropriate...the minimum that should be offered is the best intervention currently available as part of the national public health system." Or in other words, researchers are not obliged to serve as agents of change; practicality counts. Indeed, it counts so much that the standard of care that researchers must deliver is that found in the national *public* health care system, not in the private, and almost always superior, system.

All these commentaries notwithstanding, the debate on first principles not only continues but there have been several striking examples of successful opposition to placebo trials and denial of treatment. The most publicized and effective one emanated from a group of commercial sex workers in Cambodia. The research at issue was to take place in Phnom Penh as part of an NIH–CDC–Gates Foundation PREP trial, that is, pre-exposure prophylaxis in high-risk groups. The subjects were to be HIV-negative commercial sex workers; they would be given an antiretroviral drug, in this case tenofovir (Viread), and investigators would conduct follow-up studies to see whether the drug prevented the onset of HIV-AIDS. The sex workers interrupted a session at the 2004 International Aids Conference in Bangkok to protest the trial, getting international media coverage; they also convinced the Cambodian government to halt it. Their substantive points were the familiar ones: counseling of the sex workers was inadequate because researchers had an obvious stake in their continuing their high-risk behavior, and provision of medical services was inadequate for those who contracted the disease during or after the trial. From the sex workers' perspective, they were taking all the risks and getting none of the benefits.

The investigators insisted that the counseling was adequate and that all subjects would receive state-of-the-art treatment if they seroconverted during the trial, although they could not promise lifelong treatment. The responses, however, did not get the trial back on track in Cambodia. In fact, the protests then spread to Cameroon, and in February 2005, its government stopped the research. There have also been protests in Thailand, repeating some of the other objections but adding a new one: subjects who are intravenous drug users should be given clean needles along with condoms. The researchers countered that Thailand does not have a harm-reduction program and hence they were giving subjects bleach to clean used needles. But that did little to pacify the protestors.

Thus the ethics of clinical research in developing countries has moved from the pages of the *New England Journal of Medicine* to the streets, and investigators are understandably anxious. In September 2005, a group of them published a plea in *Science*: "Promote HIV Chemoprophylaxis Research, Don't Halt It." After presenting the many and undisputed reasons why a preventative for AIDS is important, they moved to the central issue in the protest: treatment for research subjects. "Community expectations for access to treatment," they wrote, "should prompt good will efforts but should not create ethical obligations that would block prevention research in locations where treatment is not available." But good will is no longer good enough. The would-be subjects of research want treatment, not promises. Investigators are going to have to do more, much more, if they are to carry on their human experiments.

4

SERVING CLIO AND CLIENT:
THE HISTORIAN AS EXPERT WITNESS

Historians in the Courtroom

THE FIRST BUT perhaps least appreciated fact about historians as expert witnesses is how often they assume the role. Although their colleagues and even litigators presume that historians rarely enter the courtroom, in fact it has been a common occurrence for some fifty years. Its origins are in the civil rights era, specifically with the case of *Brown* v. *Board of Education* (1954). Historians were not literally in that courtroom; rather, with different degrees of intellectual comfort, they helped draft the briefs presented to the Supreme Court by the lawyers for the NAACP Legal Defense and Educational Fund. In the summer of 1953, such notable historians as C. Vann Woodward, John Hope Franklin, and Alfred Kelly applied their knowledge to buttress the argument—crucial to the case—that the principle of "separate but equal" as put forward in *Plessy* v. *Ferguson* was not a neutral principle but born of a fundamental hostility toward blacks, and that Jim Crow laws represented efforts to control and humiliate the former slaves.[1] The

---

1. Richard Kluger, *Simple Justice: The History of "Brown v. Board of Education" and Black America's Struggle for Equality* (Vintage, 1975), pp. 84, 623–624, 626, 638; Paul Soifer, "The Litigation Historian: Objectivity, Responsibility, and Sources," *Public Historian*, Vol. 5, No. 2 (1983), pp. 47–62, see esp. p. 51.

historians also helped to fashion the argument that the Fourteenth and Fifteenth Amendments provided a constitutional basis for overriding the *Plessy* v. *Ferguson* precedent and shaking loose from its doctrine.[2]

The tradition born in *Brown* was maintained in a variety of other, very different cases. Historians have often testified in litigation involving Indian claims—presenting evidence, on one or the other side, as to whether the plaintiff tribe was, historically speaking, a "real" tribe; the answer had the most tangible implications for buttressing claims to particular lands or establishing native fishing and hunting rights.[3] They have also gone into court to address such questions as whether a particular river was or was not "navigable" in the nineteenth century: by offering testimony on whether a river's boat traffic was steady throughout the year (the river, therefore, to be deemed navigable) or only seasonal (and so not navigable), they helped determine whether that river fell under local or federal jurisdiction.[4] American historians have also testified in foreign courts. Salo Baron testified for the prosecution in the Israeli trial of Adolf Eichmann. The "truth" of the Holocaust took Deborah Lippstadt (in her own defense, to be sure) to England. The role of Maurice Papon in the Vichy government took Robert Paxton to France, where he testified against Papon to rebut the claim that he was merely following German orders.[5]

By far the most controversial case in the 1980s that pitted historian against historian involved charges of sexual discrimination made

2. Kluger, *Simple Justice*, pp. 291, 626, 635, 637–641, 643, 654, 668; Soifer, "Litigation Historian," pp. 51–53.

3. Heather K. Cyr, "The Battle over History," *Brunswickian*, November 4, 1999; www.unb .ca/web/bruns/9900/issue9/new/historybattle.html (May 22, 2002).

4. Carl M. Becker, "Professor for the Plaintiff: Classroom to Courtroom," *Public Historian*, Vol. 4, No. 3 (1982), pp. 69–77; Leland R. Johnson, "Public Historian for the Defendant," *Public Historian*, Vol. 5, No. 3 (1983), pp. 65–76.

5. Robert O. Paxton, "The Trial of Maurice Papon," *The New York Review of Books*, December 16, 1999, pp. 32–38.

by the Equal Employment Opportunity Commission (EEOC) against Sears, Roebuck and Company. Rosalind Rosenberg testified on behalf of Sears that the absence of women in the highest-paying sectors of its workforce represented not discrimination but an exercise of women's preferences about the kinds of jobs they wanted to do. Alice Kessler-Harris testified for the EEOC that Sears was guilty of discrimination: that it was their hiring and promotion practices, not women's choices, that shaped opportunities within the company hierarchy.[6]

In the 1990s, historians were to be found even more regularly in the courtroom. They appeared on both sides of lawsuits involving tobacco companies, answering questions regarding what was known at a given point in time about the health dangers of smoking. Kenneth Ludmerer has testified on behalf of Philip Morris. Theodore Marmor, a political scientist with a historical orientation, has also testified for tobacco companies, and so has Stephen Ambrose.[7] On the other hand, Allan Brandt is currently advising the Justice Department in its suits against tobacco companies.[8] Historians have also entered cases brought against companies based on exposure to lead and to silicosis, with David Rosner and Gerald Markowitz allied with plaintiffs.[9]

The catalog of historians in the courtroom can easily be expanded, as my own experiences amply demonstrate. I have served as a historian-expert witness on four occasions. The first case, in the 1970s, focused on the question of whether conditions of solitary confinement as then

---

6. Alice Kessler-Harris, "Equal Employment Opportunity Commission v. Sears, Roebuck and Company: A Personal Account," *Radical History Review*, Vol. 35 (1986), pp. 57–79; Rosalind Rosenberg, "Disparity or Discrimination?," interview with David Tell, *Society*, Vol. 24, No. 6 (1987), pp. 4–16; Ruth Milkman, "Women's History and the Sears Case," *Feminist Studies*, Vol. 12, No. 2 (1986), pp. 375–400.

7. Laura Maggi, "Bearing Witness for Tobacco," *American Prospect*, Vol. 11, No. 10 (2000), pp. 23–25.

8. Allan Brandt, personal communication.

9. David Rosner, personal communication.

practiced at the state prison in Walpole, Massachusetts, violated the constitutional standard of "cruel and unusual punishment." On behalf of a public interest law firm interested in prison reform, I toured the facility and then testified about both the standard itself and the conditions at the institution.

My other three cases followed on my joining the faculty at the Columbia College of Physicians and Surgeons, and all have involved the historical development of the concept of informed consent. Thus I testified for the Mental Health Law Project in its suit against the CIA for having funded, in the 1950s, the research of a Canadian psychiatrist who experimented on his patients with a technique he called "psychic driving." The CIA was interested in the possibility that the method—which forced the patient to listen to a tape playing meaningless messages repetitively and at high speeds for hours at a time—might become a tool in interrogation. In this period, US military and intelligence agencies were caught up in the possibilities of "brainwashing"—both how it might be used by others (notably China) on captured American troops and how they might use it themselves. The question for the historian in this case was: What standards of informed consent should be applied to research conducted in the 1950s? Should the psychiatrist have obtained consent from his patients before putting them through "psychic driving" (which was the plaintiffs' position), or was that requirement not yet established (the CIA stance)? For reasons to be explored later, I believed that the standard was in place. A bioethicist, Thomas Beauchamp, argued against me that it was not. The case did not go beyond the stage of depositions because the CIA decided to settle rather than litigate.[10]

I also advised one of the attorneys in a case brought by Katie Kelley Moreau. In the 1950s, in an effort to better understand the risks of radiation exposure, organs were removed from bodies that were

---

10. The case was litigated as *Orlikow v. United States*, 682 FS 77 (DDC 1988).

undergoing autopsy, sent to a Los Alamos laboratory, and never returned. The purpose of the research was to compare radioactive uptake in the organs of those who had died after working and living in the town itself with the organs of those who had worked and lived within the Los Alamos facility.[11] The issue was not whether consent for the removal of the organs had been obtained: all parties agreed that the families had given permission only for autopsy. Rather, was it necessary in the 1950s to have explicit consent for permanently removing an organ? My findings, based on an examination of discussions in pathology journals and texts, was that the need to obtain consent for removal was widely known and recognized. This case, too, was settled before trial, with the plaintiffs winning a $9 million award.

Finally, in the case that I will analyze in depth below, I testified for the plaintiffs in *Craft* v. *Vanderbilt* on the ethical standards that governed research in the years 1945 to 1960. The experiments in question involved feeding pregnant women radioactive iron in order to study its rate of absorption. The case also posed a second question, which brought in still other historians, including Robert Proctor for the plaintiffs and Susan Lindee for the defendants: What was known at that time about the risks of ingesting radioactive substances?

Let one final example demonstrate how often historians serve as expert witnesses, and how legitimate it is for them to do so. The American Historical Association in a brochure and on its Web site describes some possible nonteaching alternatives for historians. The AHA includes "Litigation Support" in its roster, counseling historians about opportunities that may be available for them to serve as expert witnesses.[12] Clearly, testifying is now considered a mainstream activity.

---

11. Dorothy Nelkin and Lori Andrews, "Do the Dead Have Interests," *American Journal of Law & Medicine*, Vol. 24, No. 23 (1998), pp. 261–291.

12. American Historical Association, "Careers in History: A Miniguide from the American Historical Association," www.theaha.org/pubs/careers/Advocate.htm (May 22, 2002).

Anxieties and Controversies

This legitimacy acknowledged, it must also be recognized that bringing Clio into the courtroom raises considerable anxiety and controversy as well, with many creditable commentators and participants worried that professional standards for scholarship cannot be fully maintained when serving as an expert witness. C. Vann Woodward was among the first to articulate the position even as he participated in the *Brown* v. *Board of Education* litigation. "I would stick to what happened and account for it as intelligently as I could," he commented. "You see I don't want to be in a position of delivering a gratuitous history lecture to the Court. And at the same time, I don't want to get out of my role as historian." The litigators were impatient with him. As one of them responded: "We wanted the historians to look at the whole thing from the viewpoint of the blacks and their aspirations, not from some cloud."[13] Alfred Kelly also shared some of Woodward's concerns, but more readily shifted roles from historian to advocate. At first he thought he could serve both masters, the discipline and the litigation—but in short order, he found himself acting more and more as a committed advocate: "I am very much afraid," he later commented, "that...I ceased to function as an historian, and instead took up the practice of law without a license." He passed this verdict on himself once he defined his assignment as an effort, not to find "the whole truth" but to convince the court that there was "something of an historical case" to overturn *Plessy* v. *Ferguson* and the separate-but-equal doctrine.[14]

More recently, Robert Paxton has expressed some of these same reservations. He had hoped that his testimony on Papon's Vichy role

---

13. Kluger, *Simple Justice*, p. 623. See also Jack Greenberg, *Crusaders in the Courts* (Basic Books, 1994), p. 188.

14. Alfred H. Kelly, "When the Supreme Court Ordered Desegregation," *US News & World Report*, February 5, 1962, pp. 86–88, quotation on p. 88.

would serve to educate the broader French public about Vichy, but he found instead that "Papon's trial could not teach the clear, simple, and unanimously agreed-upon history lesson that many advocates of the prosecution had hoped for.... Some historians doubted that historical scholarship was compatible with the procedures of a trial for crimes against humanity."[15]

If *Brown* v. *Board of Education* and the Papon trial highlight historians' anxieties, the Sears case illuminates the depths to which controversy can descend. Rosalind Rosenberg was brought into the case by one of the Sears attorneys (her ex-husband, in fact) not because of her special expertise in labor history but because she taught women's history. The EEOC was making its case on discrimination by an unusual method, relying on the statistical distribution of women in the company workforce, not on firsthand charges of unfairness. The Sears defense was that "mere" numbers did not add up to discrimination: if women were not found in the sectors that were higher paying (such as those that sold appliances), it was because of their own personal preferences. Rosenberg agreed with their contentions, arguing that discrimination was not the key to the outcome, but rather that women had agency and expressed it by preferring some jobs to others.[16]

The EEOC had not initially sought out a historian, but facing the need to rebut Rosenberg, it turned to Alice Kessler-Harris. She insisted that corporations were not nearly as passive in the process of distributing positions as Rosenberg suggested, that the messages they transmitted by dint of their own hiring record not only shaped but also coerced women's choices. Hence, statistical findings on discrimination were accurate and reliable indicators of company policy.[17]

---

15. Paxton, "The Trial of Maurice Papon," p. 38.

16. Milkman, "Women's History," p. 385; Rosenberg, "Disparity," pp. 5–6.

17. Milkman, "Women's History," p. 387; Kessler-Harris, "Equal Employment Opportunity Commission," pp. 66–72.

The federal court ruled for Sears. In fact, its decision noted specifically that it found Rosenberg's approach far more compelling than Kessler-Harris's.[18] In short order, a bitter debate broke out about Rosenberg's role in the case, with Kessler-Harris and many other women historians taking a very critical stance. Some of the controversy involved whether Rosenberg, who often cited Kessler-Harris's research in her own depositions, had misused her scholarship. But the nub of the issue, certainly to Kessler-Harris, was political: Why would a feminist historian go to work for Sears, help them in their case, and set back the cause of women's economic advancement? Writing in 1986 in the *Radical History Review*, Kessler-Harris declared: "It did not surprise me that history was brought to trial.... But I continue to be disturbed that a feminist historian should fail to see the implications of her testimony for working women and for women's history."[19]

With historians voting, as it were, with their feet and regularly entering the courtroom, it becomes all the more critical to consider the implications of this activity for the standards of the craft. Are those standards inevitably compromised when historians occupy the witness chair? Can you do justice to history even as you try to obtain justice for plaintiff or defendant?

In an effort to answer these questions, I will focus on the case of *Craft* v. *Vanderbilt*, but in a very special way. In the first instance, I will describe my research and writing activities for the plaintiffs: what I did and did not do in addressing the questions of ethics and the history of human experimentation in my capacity as expert witness. But then, in the second instance, I will describe my research and writing activities in preparation for the Garrison Lecture of 2002: what I did and did not do in addressing these very same questions for another audience. The occasion of the Garrison Lecture serves as a test case

---

18. Milkman, "Women's History," pp. 390–391.

19. Kessler-Harris, "Equal Employment Opportunity Commission," p. 75.

for me. I return to the same story, but this time so as to enlighten my professional colleagues, not lawyers and judges. The differences between the two performances—and there are differences—are what I wish to emphasize, using them as the springboard for conclusions about serving Clio and serving clients.

Serving the Client

Between 1945 and 1949, some 830 to 850 pregnant women using the Vanderbilt University prenatal clinic were fed single doses of iron tagged with a radioactive isotope on their second visit.[20] The purpose of the dose was to enable investigators, notably William Darby and Paul Hahn, to learn about iron absorption in pregnant women so as to calculate the amount of iron they needed and to establish the most effective regimen for delivering it. Although there is some dispute about what the investigators actually said to the women, the women themselves remember being told that the dose was a "vitamin cocktail"—and the record supports them. In any event, the Vanderbilt defense was not that Darby and Hahn had obtained informed consent, but rather that the principle itself was not yet embedded in research practice. The plaintiffs, for their part, insisted not only that consent was necessary and appropriate, but that the Vanderbilt team had practiced outright deception.

In 1969 another Vanderbilt team, headed by Ruth Hagstrom, conducted a follow-up study of the health of the women who had participated in the original research. Relying on a detailed questionnaire, the purpose of the study was "to determine morbidity and mortality

---

20. P. F. Hahn, E. L. Carothers, et al., "Iron Metabolism in Human Pregnancy as Studied with the Radioactive Isotope, Fe59," *American Journal of Obstetrics and Gynecology*, Vol. 61, No. 3 (1951), pp. 477–486.

experiences in the children and mothers fed radioactive iron." The Hagstrom study was stimulated by findings that postnatal exposure to radiation in other instances had caused "an increased incidence of leukemia and other malignancies in both children and adults."[21] Would this also be true for the Vanderbilt women and their children?

None of this background information, however, was shared with the recipients of the questionnaires. They were not told why the study was being conducted. Nor were they told that as participants in the 1945–1949 research they had been fed radioactive iron. Instead, they were addressed as those who had earlier joined a "diet and eating habits" study and were then asked about the state of their and their children's health.

The Hagstrom investigation succeeded in reaching some 90 percent of the original cohort. It found that, compared to a control group, the research group demonstrated "a small but significant increase" in cancer rates among their children—namely, three cases of cancers linked to radioactive substances among 654 children.[22] The findings were published in the *American Journal of Epidemiology*, but neither the women nor the children were told about them.

The story lay dormant—not hidden, because the articles were in the literature for anyone to read—until the sudden turn of attention to radiation experiments following the Pulitzer Prize–winning reporting of Eileen Welsome, a New Mexico journalist. With cold war mentalities receding, and under significant public pressure, Secretary of Energy Hazel O'Leary ordered the release of previously classified materials about radiation experiments, in the process creating a

---

21. Ruth M. Hagstrom, S. R. Glasser, et al., "Long Term Effects of Radioactive Iron Administered during Human Pregnancy," *American Journal of Epidemiology*, Vol. 90, No. 1 (1969), pp. 1–10, quotation on p. 2.

22. Ruth Hagstrom, Transcript of February 16, 1997, Deposition, *Craft* v. *Vanderbilt*, M. D. Tenn. Docket no. 3-94-0090, on pp. 120–122.

remarkable archive.[23] As a result, litigators learned about the Vanderbilt research, contacted the women involved, and organized a class action lawsuit: *Emma Craft* v. *Vanderbilt* (also including as a defendant the Rockefeller Foundation, which had funded the research). The women were seeking monetary damages and an apology.

The law firm that brought the case, Lief, Cabraser, Heimann & Bernstein, based in San Francisco, was not a public interest law firm but a highly successful litigating group that reaped significant profits from the class action suits that it won. One of their attorneys, Donald Arbitblitt, telephoned me and efficiently laid out the reason for his call: Vanderbilt and Rockefeller were claiming that there was no need in the 1945–1949 period to obtain informed consent for research. Arbitblitt had already read what I had written about the history of human experimentation, including my *New England Journal of Medicine* analysis of Henry Beecher's 1966 exposé of research protocols of dubious ethicality and *Strangers at the Bedside*.[24] He was therefore able to phrase his question to me very succinctly: Would I be willing to testify that ethical standards in the 1945–1949 period were such that defendants violated them by not obtaining consent? I readily accepted—but let me leave the reasons for later discussion.

What did I receive? The boxes that arrived included depositions from Darby, Hagstrom, and others (Hahn had already died), along with reports and depositions from plaintiffs' experts. There were also relevant documents drawn from the Rockefeller Foundation archives, describing research activities proposed and to be conducted, and

---

23. Eileen Welsome, *The Plutonium Files: America's Secret Medical Experiments in the Cold War* (Delacorte, 1999).

24. David Rothman, "Ethics and Human Experimentation: Henry Beecher Revisited," *New England Journal of Medicine*, Vol. 317 (1987), pp. 1195–1199; Henry Beecher, *Strangers at the Bedside: A History of How Law and Bioethics Transformed Medical Decision Making* (Basic Books, 1991).

internal memos from the Vanderbilt investigators and administrators obtained under legal rules governing "discovery" of evidence. If an article or reference struck me as important, the law firm would obtain it for me, readily serving as research assistant. I was to read all this and anything else I believed relevant—billing the firm at the rate of several hundred dollars an hour—and ultimately to produce a report laying out my position, a rebuttal to their expert's report; to undergo a deposition; and, if needed, to appear as a witness in court.

The question posed was straightforward: What were the ethical standards that researchers in 1945–1949 were obliged to respect? Vanderbilt contended that there were no existing state or federal statutes governing the conduct of human experimentation that mandated consent. Moreover, principles of consent at this time were neither taught formally in medical schools nor transmitted informally from physician or investigator to students. Most important, in practice, investigators did not routinely ask subjects for consent to perform research on them, particularly when the subjects were also patients. To substantiate the point, Vanderbilt cited Henry Beecher's 1966 article and *Strangers at the Bedside*, both of which documented instances in which researchers had failed to obtain consent. Finally, Vanderbilt brought in Robert Levine—professor of medicine at Yale, editor of a newsletter, *IRB*, and a frequent writer and commentator on the ethics of research—to support its contentions. Levine corroborated their position, arguing that since the women were patients at the clinic, it was not necessary to obtain their consent.[25]

From my perspective, Vanderbilt had it wrong. It was elevating the practice of some, even many, investigators to constitute a standard for all: because they had not obtained consent, it was therefore right not to obtain consent. But the fact that a principle was flouted does not

---

25. Robert Levine, Transcript of September 17, 1997, Deposition, *Craft* v. *Vanderbilt*, on pp. 258–261.

mean that the principle was not operative. Accordingly, I focused my analysis on the normative statements that were relevant to the ethics of research, and presented a very different picture.

In the first instance, I argued that concepts of bodily integrity were relevant to the ethics of experimentation. It was well appreciated long before the 1970s that no one, including researchers, had the right to violate bodily integrity without explicit permission—whether the act was a physical assault, a surgical procedure, an injection, or, as in this case, an iron supplement tagged with a radioactive substance. I referred, as would be expected, to Benjamin Cardozo's classic decision in *Schloendorff v. Society of New York Hospital* (1914): "Every human being of adult years and sound mind has a right to determine what shall be done with his own body; and a surgeon who performs an operation without his patient's consent commits an assault for which he is liable in damages."[26] If this principle governed medical care, surely it governed research; and if it were true for 1914, surely it was true for 1945 as well. In this same spirit, I noted that medicine for centuries had reiterated the ideal of "do no harm," an injunction that was certainly no less relevant to research than to therapeutics. The physician's obligation is to promote the well-being of the patient, not to put the patient at risk, even if the precise level of the risk can be debated.

From arguments by extension I moved next to explore the principles that addressed human experimentation directly, uncovering an intricate and detailed record of commentary, almost all of which confirmed the need for consent prior to research. This review of the normative statements occupied center stage in my report. I argued that

> the standards applicable to research in the period 1945–1947 included informing the subjects in an experiment that they were participating in a research protocol, making certain that they

---

26. *Schloendorff v. Society of New York Hospital*, 211 NY 125, 105 NE 92, 93 (1914).

understood its components, and obtaining their consent to participate in the research. Although the standards for research with a therapeutic potential were somewhat more ambiguous, there is no doubt that these enumerated standards were clearly applicable to research with no potential therapeutic benefit to the subjects. Feeding radioactive iron to human subjects represents a manifest example of non-therapeutic research, and as such, the investigators were ethically required to inform the subjects of the fact of the experiment, the details of the experiment, the risks of the experiment, and obtain their consent to participate.[27]

In support of these propositions, I invoked texts both well known and more obscure. I quoted Claude Bernard, writing in 1865 in *An Introduction to the Study of Experimental Medicine*. Bernard fully appreciated the importance of clinical research, designating it the third pillar of medical knowledge. Even so, he insisted that investigators were never entitled to sacrifice the interests of the subject for the benefit of others:

> Experiments, then, may be performed on man, but within what limits? It is our duty and our right to perform an experiment on man whenever it can save his life, cure him or gain him some personal benefit. The principle of medical and surgical morality, therefore, consists in never performing on man an experiment which might be harmful to him to any extent, even though the result might be highly advantageous to science, i.e., to the health of others.[28]

---

27. David J. Rothman, Statement of Expert Witness, *Craft v. Vanderbilt*, p. 6.

28. Claude Bernard, *An Introduction to the Study of Experimental Medicine*, translated by Henry C. Greene (MacMillan, 1927), pp. 101–102.

I went on to observe that some forty years later, in 1907, these same principles were repeated and expanded by the eminent Johns Hopkins professor of medicine William Osler. He not only condemned harmful nontherapeutic research (as did Bernard), but insisted that the principle of consent of the subject had to govern the research:

> For man absolute safety and full consent are the conditions which make such tests allowable. We have no right to use patients entrusted to our care for the purpose of experimentation unless direct benefit to the individual is likely to follow. Once this limit is transgressed, the sacred cord which binds physician and patient snaps instantly.[29]

In effect, Osler enunciated the principles of consent well in advance of the Nuremberg Code.

The viewpoints expressed by Bernard and Osler, I contended, were shared widely. In 1886, as Susan Lederer's history of early human experimentation explained, a Boston physician, Charles Francis Withington, published an essay entitled "The Relation of Hospitals to Medical Education," which won Harvard's prestigious Boylston Prize. Withington posed the question of research ethics in terms of the "possible conflict between the interests of medical science and those of the individual patient, and the latter's indefeasible rights," and he came down staunchly on the side of patient rights, even to the point of suggesting, as a remedy, a patients' "Bill of Rights":

> In the older countries of Europe especially, where the life and happiness of the so-called lower classes are perhaps held more cheaply than with us, enthusiastic devotees of science are very

---

29. William Osler, "The Evolution of the Idea of Experiment in Medicine," *Transcripts of the Congress of American Physicians & Surgeons*, Vol. 7 (1907), pp. 1–8, quotation on pp. 7–8.

apt to encroach upon the rights of the individual patient in a manner which cannot be justified. In this country, we are less likely to fall into this error than those living under monarchical institutions, but even with us it may be well to draw up, as it were, a Bill of Rights which shall secure patients against any injustice from the votaries of science.[30]

Withington insisted that patients had "a right to immunity from experiments merely as such, and outside the therapeutic application. This right is one that is especially liable to violation by enthusiastic investigators." Investigators who wanted to examine the potency of a new drug had to rely upon volunteers, but "they had no right to make any man the unwilling victim of such an experiment." Withington concluded with a sentence that encapsulated the core ethical principle: "The occupants of hospital wards are something more than merely so much clinical material during their lives and so much pathological material after their death."[31]

In light of the Vanderbilt contentions, I demonstrated that these principles were invoked to chastise a particular investigator who violated them. Osler condemned a protocol that involved the purposeful infection of subjects, without obtaining their permission, with what researchers believed to be the bacillus responsible for yellow fever: "To deliberately inject a poison of known high degree of virulency into a human being, unless you obtain that man's sanction, is not ridiculous, it is criminal."[32] In these same terms, Osler, along with

30. Charles Francis Withington, *The Relation of Hospitals to Medical Education* (Cupples, Upham, 1886), p. 5. See also Susan E. Lederer, *Subjected to Science: Human Experimentation in America Before the Second World War* (Oxford University Press, 1995).

31. Withington, *The Relation of Hospitals to Medical Education*, pp. 15–17.

32. William Osler, discussion of George M. Sternberg, "The Bacillus Icteroides (Sanarelli) and Bacillus X (Sternberg)," *Trans. Assoc. Amer. Physicians*, Vol. 13 (1898), p. 71.

many colleagues, condemned the cancer research conducted by two German surgeons who transplanted malignant cells from the diseased breast of a patient to her second, healthy breast in order to study the transmissibility of cancer cells.[33] Commenting on the research, the *Journal of the American Medical Association* endorsed the refusal of a French medical academy to allow a discussion of the medical implications of the findings because they had been obtained in so unethical a fashion. *JAMA* itself hoped that "the storm of indignation which has been aroused, shall deter others who might have in view, in their zeal for science, similar unjustifiable experiments."[34]

The Nuremberg Code, I argued, was not invented out of thin air so as to find a means to punish German doctors. Promulgated in 1947, it emphasized the need for informed consent. As its very first principle put it:

> The voluntary consent of the human subject is absolutely essential. This means the person involved should have legal capacity to give consent... and should have sufficient knowledge and comprehension of the elements of the subject matter involved so as to enable him to make an understanding and enlightened decision.[35]

From my perspective, Nuremberg was invoking an already well-established position, not subjecting German perpetrators to ex post facto judgments.

I went on to insist that not only had the original iron research violated known and recognized standards but so did, in even more

33. Cited in Lederer, *Subjected to Science*, p. 63.

34. "Grafting Cancer in the Human Subject," *Journal of the American Medical Association*, Vol. 17 (1891), pp. 233–234, quotation on p. 234.

35. *The Nazi Doctors and the Nuremberg Code*, edited by George J. Annas and Michael A. Grodin (Oxford University Press, 1992), pp. 102–103.

egregious fashion, Hagstrom's follow-up study. By 1969, when she published her findings, Beecher's work had already appeared and discussions of consent requirements were frequently found in the literature. Moreover, in 1964 the World Medical Association had promulgated its Declaration of Helsinki, with its unambiguous insistence that subjects of research must be informed of its aims, methods, benefits, and hazards before they participated. Surely, then, the Hagstrom team had an ethical obligation to inform the subjects why they were being contacted and the nature of the risk to which they had been exposed. Any possible doubt about the importance of fulfilling this duty was erased by the fact that the team had found "a small, but statistically significant increase"[36] in malignancies among the children, an increase that they believed "suggests a cause and effect relationship." Hagstrom insisted that informing the subjects of the results of the follow-up would have needlessly "alarmed" them and "doesn't make sense."[37] But it was the subject's prerogative, not the investigator's, to determine what risk is worth worrying about.

The Vanderbilt lawyers—ever so competent, well versed in the materials, and familiar with all of my relevant writings—were not without countervailing arguments. They asked me who had read Bernard and Osler, and how I could be certain that their views were known and accepted. Again and again they returned to the violations in practice that my own research had uncovered, insisting that practice indicated an absence of principle. My responses emphasized the extraordinary regard in which Bernard and Osler were held, the high degree of consistency among the commentators, and, with all due repetition, that transgressions do not invalidate principles.

There never was the occasion to argue all this out before a jury: Vanderbilt and Rockefeller settled the case with a $10 million payout

---

36. Hagstrom, Glasser et al., "Long Term Effects," p. 1.

37. Hagstrom Deposition, p. 121; see also pp. 66, 104, 120–121, 128.

and an apology. When their lawyer began to read the apology to the judge, he was told to turn around, face the plaintiffs, and read it to them.

Serving Clio

Inspired by the invitation to deliver the Garrison Lecture, I returned to the Vanderbilt research—this time not to serve as an expert witness in a case but to analyze the events as the basis for a lecture to colleagues and for a scholarly article. No sooner did I undertake this assignment than I found myself opening wide the door of inquiry, going well beyond what had been my focus for the court case into a series of fascinating issues that I had not explored before. I was now far less concerned with who was right and who was wrong than I was with how it happened that Vanderbilt undertook this research; what frame of mind, ethics aside, the investigators brought to the work; how it related to other ongoing investigations; why Rockefeller funded it; and so on. As soon as I was a historian in the archive, not in the courtroom, instinctively and reflexively I broadened the scope of inquiry. I moved, in photographic terms, from a narrow and tight shot to a wide angle. I had a different lens on my camera, and it brought into focus a whole range of new considerations.

A few examples easily establish the differences. In my historian's role, I had a special interest in the composition of the Vanderbilt subjects. I suspected that many people who had read brief newspaper accounts of the study presumed that since the research was risky and no consent was obtained, the subjects had to be African-Americans living in Tennessee. In fact, every one of the subjects was white. Why was this so? The answer turns out to be very simple: Vanderbilt's prenatal clinic was segregated, serving whites only; the blacks went to Meharry. That fact had never come up in my conversations with the plaintiffs or in questioning from the defendants. Apparently, neither side found it a useful piece of information. The defendants were not about to claim that if the research had been truly dangerous it would not have been performed on whites, and the plaintiffs saw no reason to emphasize the whiteness of the class. But every historian, to understate the point, would consider this a useful piece of information, perhaps even the first item on the research agenda. Was Vanderbilt another Tuskegee? Was there a racial component to the research? Was this yet another example of white physicians putting black subjects at risk? That these most elemental historical questions were altogether absent from the court record stands as a perfect example of the difference between the perspective of a case and the perspective of a discipline.

By the same token, the question of why Vanderbilt undertook research into iron absorption was of minor interest to the litigating parties but of central interest to a historical inquiry. It turns out that in a fuller analysis of the incident, the changing grant policies of the Rockefeller Foundation assume special importance: in this period, it was altering its philanthropy from endowing a few promising academic institutions to supporting specific studies by investigators wherever they might be found. Vanderbilt was caught in the middle of this change and, in response, began to undertake specific research projects as a source of funding for personnel and facilities. Already in 1945–1949, skills at grant-getting had assumed significance. Paul Hahn was appointed to the Vanderbilt department of chemistry but he was junior in rank, in need of salary support, and obliged to design and carry out research that would attract funding. William Darby was trying to build up a division of nutrition at Vanderbilt and recognized that he would accomplish the task only through outside support. In all, it was apparent by 1946 that "soft money" was essential to university-based research. As one noted Vanderbilt investigator, writing in *Science*, explained: "The universities must be provided with large sums of money for education, research, and training, as free as possible of restrictions.... The conduct of research [is] really the highest form of teaching." Hence "medical research...has a pre-eminent call upon every social structure for support.... Let each social order give the scientist a free hand." Give him the environment and the tools he needs for his research, "and otherwise, for humanity's sake, leave him alone."[38]

But it was not grantsmanship alone that drove the research forward. The field of human nutrition was undergoing major development during these years, partly as a result of the recent discovery of the role of vitamins. As yet, very little was known about their contributions to human health. That vitamin deficiencies had a distinctive role in causing some diseases was appreciated, but the relation of vitamins to general physical and mental well-being was just being explored. The interest was high, and the potential results important. Indeed, investigators at Vanderbilt and elsewhere were eager to learn more not only about iron uptake in pregnant women but also about the general nutritional states of whites and blacks in Tennessee, hoping that their findings would enable them to raise the levels of health in both groups. However well-intentioned the motives, the plaintiffs in the court case were altogether uninterested in the scientific bases for the research, and the defendants, too, found them irrelevant. To historians, however, they are among the most critical elements in the story.

Perhaps the most astonishing result of casting a wider net of inquiry came where I expected it least: in the history of human experimentation in mental hospitals. Although I certainly knew a good deal about this subject, I was unaware of the history of vitamin research at the Elgin State Hospital in Illinois. How did I happen upon this material? Again, the wide angle is critical. In order to better understand why Vanderbilt was so interested in vitamin research, I looked

---

38. Ernest W. Goodpasture, "Research and Medical Practice," *Science*, Vol. 104 (1946), pp. 473–476.

into its other sources of funding and came upon the Nutrition Institute, itself supported by a number of major food companies. Reading more about the institute, I learned of its support of Vanderbilt, but then, to my astonishment, learned also about its support for investigators at the Elgin State Hospital. Once I was put on track, the rest was easy. The annual reports of the hospital itself and the articles that appeared in the medical journals on the results of the research told the story fully—and what a story it was.[39]

I might have anticipated it. After all, the broader my inquiry, the more I learned about other highly invasive research activities with radioactive substances that the Vanderbilt investigators had carried out. In 1943, Paul Hahn reported in the *American Journal of Obstetrics and Gynecology* a study of rates of absorption of radioactive sodium into the vaginas of seven women. The women were not identified, but they were described as having just delivered a baby or undergone surgery, and thus, in the investigator's language, had a "traumatized vagina." The article went on to explain that in order "to prevent leakage, the subjects' hips were slightly elevated and a small cotton tampon inserted just within the vaginal outlet. Blood samples were then taken at frequent intervals from the cubital veins."[40] The result of the research was a better understanding of vaginal absorption and recommendations to be particularly cautious about using toxic ingredients as a douche. But whether the women had volunteered for the study, or even been told that they were in a study, was not mentioned. Invoking one of Henry Beecher's principles, it is most likely that given the discomfort, pain, and danger of the research, the subjects did not knowingly and willingly consent to it.

---

39. Charles Glen King, *A Good Idea: The History of the Nutrition Foundation* (Nutrition Foundation, 1976), pp. 223–228.

40. W. T. Pommerenke and P. F. Hahn, "Absorption of Radioactive Sodium Instilled into the Vagina," *American Journal of Obstetrics and Gynecology*, Vol. 46 (1943), pp. 853–855.

The research conducted at Elgin, which was still more invasive and would not pass the test of informed consent, represented a collaboration between the Food and Nutrition Board of the National Research Council and the Elgin State Hospital. It was also supported by the Milbank Foundation and by the Macy Foundation. The initiative came from Dr. M. K. Horwitt, who was director of the Biochemical Research Laboratory of the hospital, running a small research wing that, in 1942, was eager to study metabolism in schizophrenics.[41] Horwitt, with outside support, was able to take over a one-story building on the hospital grounds and to expand the research agenda to include general vitamin requirements and the effects of vitamin deficiencies—or, as the team put it, "to attempt to create and study pure riboflavin [vitamin] deficiency in controlled circumstances."[42]

One of the first investigations—which was typical, in its method and types of findings, of other Elgin research—was published in 1948 in the *American Journal of Psychiatry*. The researchers selected three groups of twelve men each from the hospital population (the younger men were schizophrenic; the older were demented), and fed them special diets: one was deficient in vitamins B1 and B2, one was rich in these vitamins, and one was the normal hospital diet. The men were kept on the diet for two years, enabling the investigators to report that the vitamin-deficient group

> showed a general dulling of affect, loss of interest and ambition, accompanied by a decrease of motor activity.... One could see the subjects of the A [vitamin-deprived] group sitting quietly on their chairs or lying on their beds while most of the other group were moving around, helping in the ward work, talking to each

---

41. King, *A Good Idea*, p. 224.

42. O. W. Hills, E. Libert, et al., "Clinical Aspects of Dietary Depletion of Riboflavin," *Archives of Internal Medicine*, Vol. 87 (1951), pp. 682–693, quotation on p. 682.

other or reading. One elderly man who had been known always to be quick, alert, and helpful withdrew from all his activities, isolated himself, and became disinterested in his surroundings.[43]

In light of these findings, the investigators took the B group, which had been fed a vitamin-rich diet, and reduced their B_1/B_2 intake even more drastically than that of the A group. The results were even more extreme behavioral disorders. One elderly man, heretofore mildly depressed, became more deeply depressed; one mild-mannered man became violent, threatening to break furniture and escape. One of the younger men, who had heretofore easily suppressed bursts of temper, now "went into blind rages"; he became uncontrollable, "threw heavy objects at persons within his reach, screamed at the top of his lungs and cursed female attendants." On the basis of these findings, the team concluded: "Vitamin B complex restrictions caused severe primary mental changes or aggravation of pre-existing psychotic trends among the psychotic subjects."

The researchers continued their projects in order to explore the physical consequences of vitamin deprivation. In 1949, they reported in the *Journal of Nutrition* the case histories of thirteen men who had been on a vitamin B_2–deprived diet over the course of two years: within four months, one subject had lesions and fissures, a second subject had severe scrotal dermatitis, and a third suffered the "most severe" changes, including "raw and weeping" scrotal lesions, extending to the thighs.[44] The team also used the residents of Elgin to investigate niacin and protein deficiencies, in the process discovering cases

---

43. Oscar Kreisler, Erich Liebert, and M. K. Horwitt, "Psychiatric Observations on Induced Vitamin B Complex Deficiency in Psychotic Patients," *American Journal of Psychiatry*, Vol. 105 (1948), pp. 107–110.

44. M. K. Horwitt, O. W. Hills, et al., "Effects of Dietary Depletion of Riboflavin," *Journal of Nutrition*, Vol. 39 (1949), pp. 357–373, quotation on p. 368.

of liver dysfunction after five months. They were curious as well about the effects of vitamin B2 deficiency on skin sensitivity to ultra-violet exposure. As they wrote: "The fore-arms of several of the subjects were exposed to infra-red light and although small third-degree burns were inadvertently produced in three subjects, no resultant adjacent dermatitis occurred."[45]

In all, what a chapter this was in the history of mental hospitals and human experimentation—but only in my role as historian did I get to uncover it.

Conclusion

Although the distinctions I am drawing between the role of historian in the courtroom and the role of historian in the archive might seem somewhat artificial—nothing, for example, prevented me from expanding my research in preparing my report to the court, and some litigation might encourage the historian to cast the net of research more widely—in fact, they are not. At a minimum, bifurcating the roles as I do provides two ideal types for analysis and in this way helps clarify the crucial differences between the courtroom and the archive. At best, this division highlights the essential characteristics of each activity. Lawyers and judges, typically, would find the broader issues irrelevant and inadmissible. Historians would be impatient with so restricted an angle of vision.

What conclusions, then, may be drawn from my two experiences? For one, the integrity and soundness of my testimony remained. The added research that I conducted did not alter any of the findings that I had offered in my reports and depositions in the Vanderbilt case. To

---

45. M. K. Horwitt, C. C. Harvey, et al., "Tryptophan-Niacin Relationships in Man," *Journal of Nutrition*, Vol. 60, Suppl. 1 (1956), pp. 1–43, quotation on p. 13; see also p. 6.

focus an inquiry does not distort the results. Expert witnesses are not necessarily manipulating evidence to serve a client. They dare not contradict their prior positions—if they did, opposing counsel would immediately pounce on them. Indeed, to charge that expert witnesses are too committed to their side of the case to remain objective is far too simplistic. Historians are no more or less "objective" in the courtroom than they are in the lecture hall or in print.

For another, my return to the sources confirmed how very different it was to serve the client than to serve Clio. To enter the courtroom is to do many things, but it is not to do history. The essential attributes that we treasure most about historical inquiry have to be left outside the door. The scope of analysis is narrowed, the imagination is constrained, and the curiosity curtailed.

Which brings us to the final consideration: Why enter the courtroom at all? I think it is for one of two reasons. First, historians may find it important to buttress the operation of the legal system. All defendants and plaintiffs should have access to expert opinion, just as they should have access to counsel. They are entitled to their day in court, and historians, as good citizens, should help them present their most accurate case. In this sense, the historian who testifies for an unpopular client is no different from a lawyer who defends an unpopular client.

Second, historians, like other citizens, may wish to bring their expertise to the support of a cause, to seek to bring justice to a person or to groups that, in their view, have been injured or wronged. In this effort, they serve as advocates and agents of change and their justifications, I believe, should recognize this fact. For myself, serving as an expert witness represents a declaration of sympathy for those pressing the case, for the cause they represent, for the equity they wish to achieve, and for the positions they want to protect or realize. Some judges, and perhaps some colleagues as well, may prefer to think of expert witnesses as purely neutral and without personal commitment to the outcome. Such a stance, however, is not only unrealistic but also misguided. Advocacy has its place, and it can be promoted without compromising the historian's craft.

III

Rights to Equity and Fairness
in Health Care

5

RATIONING LIFE

MUST HEALTH CARE be rationed? The issue is as salient today as it was when this review appeared in 1992 and the arguments advanced then are substantially the same as those offered now. Medical schools and research centers are still holding conferences on such questions as "Is rationing inevitable?" and many commentators continue to address the question posed by the philosopher John Kilner in his book *Who Lives? Who Dies?* The inquiries are usually of three kinds. One addresses the narrow issue of which patient should get the last available bed in the intensive care unit, or the single available donated heart, or the only remaining respirator. The dilemma arises over whether to choose the candidate who is first in line, the youngest, the most prominent, or the richest, to name only some of the criteria that may be used.

A second kind of inquiry addresses the broader problem of what percentage of national resources should be devoted to health care as compared to, say, education, defense, or highway construction. The total amount of money spent annually by the government, insurance companies, and private citizens on medical care now amounts to almost $2 trillion, up from $700 billion when this article first appeared. What social choices have to be made if American medicine is to live within this already enormous budget? It is not unusual for commentators to confuse this question with the first.

The third question is to what degree health care can be distributed more equitably—not, as now, largely according to income but according to need. With 45 million people uninsured, and almost as many underinsured, those with low incomes must settle for second-rate medical care, or none at all. Were we ever to have a national health insurance system, which still does not seem likely, there would have to be some type of rationing. As one critic has noted, it is simply not possible to give everyone everything in medicine.[1]

The use of the word "rationing" has helped, at least, to begin a dialogue on the social values implicit in determining who will get effective treatment and who will not. In fact this may be why philosophers and bioethicists concerned with the moral implications of medical decisions have become prominent in a debate that might otherwise have been monopolized by political scientists, economists, and health specialists. Two much-discussed cases suggest the central ethical issues that continue to be perplexing. The first occurred in the early 1960s in Seattle, when a committee of laypeople was given the authority to decide which applicants should be able to use a kidney dialysis machine. The second took place in Oregon, where the state legislature was charged with deciding the range of medical services that would be made available to people who receive Medicaid.

In 1962, Dr. Belding Scribner of the University of Washington Medical School perfected an ingenious device to keep alive patients who would otherwise die from chronic kidney disease. They were connected to the machine by a shunt implanted in the arm between an artery and a vein; during six- to eight-hour sessions three times a week, their blood circulated through artificial filters and was cleansed of virtually all impurities.

---

1. George Lundberg, "National Health Care Reform: An Aura of Inevitability Is Upon Us," *Journal of the American Medical Association*, Vol. 265 (May 15, 1991), pp. 2566–2567.

Initially, dialysis machines were in very short supply and the people who could benefit from them far outnumbered those who could be treated. To select among the applicants, that is, to decide who would live and who would die, the Seattle medical society and the hospital appointed a committee of seven citizens who had no special qualifications—the first group was composed of a lawyer, a minister, a housewife, a labor leader, a state official, a banker, and a surgeon. A medical team first screened the patients to see if they would benefit from dialysis and the committee then decided which of the remaining candidates would receive treatment.[2]

The committee's deliberations were described in a *Life* magazine article by Shana Alexander. Having attended its meetings, she reported how members relied upon highly conventional standards. They chose married men with children over unmarried men and women, and over childless couples as well; they selected the employed over the unemployed. They rewarded "public service," giving preference to community volunteers and churchgoers. They rejected out of hand anyone who was considered deviant, whether because of a mental disability or a criminal record.

This use of narrow middle-class standards to discriminate among patients provoked a great many reactions that were highly critical of the principles the committee had adopted. "What is meant by 'public service'?" the authors of a *UCLA Law Review* article asked. "Were the persons who got themselves jailed in the South while working for civil rights doing a 'public service'? What about working for the Anti-vivisection League?" With ample justification they concluded: "The Pacific Northwest is no place for a Henry David Thoreau with bad kidneys."[3]

---

2. The first life-saving medical machine was actually the iron lung, but the relative ease of manufacture and the extraordinary fund-raising efforts of the National Foundation for Infantile Paralysis made it unnecessary to ration the use of the machine.

3. David Sanders and Jessie Dukeminier, "Medical Advance and Legal Lag: Hemiodyalysis and Kidney Transplantation," *UCLA Law Review*, Vol. 15 (1968), pp. 357–413; Renee C. Fox and Judith P. Swazey, *The Courage to Fail* (University of Chicago Press, 1974), Chapter 8.

In reaction to what had happened in Seattle, Indiana's then Senator Vance Hartke urged Congress to enact federal legislation to underwrite the entire cost of dialysis for everyone who would need it. "Tens of billions of dollars," he said, "are spent on...cosmetics to make us look pleasing, and on appliances to make our lives easier.... We can begin to set our national priorities through a national effort to bring kidney disease treatment within the reach of all those in need." Henry Jackson, the senator from Washington, made an identical case: "I think it is a great tragedy, in a nation as affluent as ours, that we have to consciously make a decision as to the people who will live and the people who will die. We had a committee in Seattle...who had to pass judgment on who would live and who would die. I believe we can do better than that."[4]

The result was a federal program that since 1973 has provided unlimited coverage to all persons suffering from life-threatening kidney disease. The current cost is approximately $16 billion a year to treat approximately 360,000 patients. (In 1992, the comparable numbers were $3 billion for 150,000.) Rather than address the question of rationing—the specific problem of who gets on the dialysis machine—Congress made an unlimited appropriation to treat kidney disease.

The conclusion shared by three specialists in bioethics who have published books on rationing is that the precedent of dialysis cannot, and should not, be followed. John Kilner, a philosopher who teaches at Trinity International University in Illinois, begins *Who Lives? Who Dies?* by discounting the "popular myth" that Americans have enough resources to underwrite the cost of treating every terminal disease.[5] Practically all new medical technologies will at first be scarce, he writes, and therefore philosophers should try to state the principles that should

4. *Congressional Record*, September 30, 1972, pp. 33,004–33,008.

5. *Who Lives? Who Dies?: Ethical Criteria in Patient Selection* (Yale University Press, 1990).

guide rationing, at least for a limited period. Paul Menzel argues in *Strong Medicine* that there is an even broader but no less inescapable conflict between the well-being of the individual patient and what he describes as the social pressures for "economic efficiency."[6] A philosopher who taught at Pacific Lutheran University, he never defines what he means by economic efficiency or who expresses its values, but he concludes nevertheless:

> Efficiency will sooner or later call for restricting care that would benefit individual patients. This is "hard efficiency": it is surely not just the elimination of waste.

He wants doctors to meet the standards of financial efficiency, even if the result is "distasteful medicine to swallow."

Daniel Callahan, a philosopher who recently retired as the director of the Hastings Center, is enthusiastic about the prospect of rationing. In *What Kind of Life*, he claims that "the financial crisis facing the healthcare system provides a superb, if probably painful, occasion to ask some basic questions once again about health and human life."[7]

The readiness of these writers to accept and promote rationing reflects a major shift in perspective among specialists in bioethics, many of whom said in the 1960s and 1970s that their primary goal was the protection of individual rights of patients against the paternalism of the physician or the state. Thus bioethicists such as Callahan led the movement to promote informed consent by patients, to force doctors to be truthful in giving a grim diagnosis, and to strengthen the patient's right to refuse treatment in both private and public hospitals. To judge by a number of recent books, concerns about collective well-being have become more important than individual rights. Callahan

---

6. *Strong Medicine: The Ethical Rationing of Health Care* (Oxford University Press, 1990).

7. *What Kind of Life: The Limits of Medical Progress* (Simon and Schuster, 1990).

insists that health care programs should be "fostering the common good and collective health of society, not the particularized good of individuals."

But any attempt to justify rationing by such concepts of collective well-being is not only exceptionally difficult but has enormous potential for mischief. In a summary of practically all the different principles that experts have suggested for allocating scarce resources to one patient rather than another, Kilner mentions social worth (as with the Seattle committee), being a member of a favored group (nationals ought to receive benefits before foreigners), imminent death (the patient about to die should have priority over the very sick patient who has, say, a year to live), as well as age, the ability to pay, and, finally, the simple principle of first-come, first-served. Kilner rather mechanically outlines the justifications and weaknesses of each; it turns out that the standards most difficult to defend on ethical grounds are, in fact, often the ones most frequently used in day-to-day practice. One obvious example is ability to pay—patients die regularly because they cannot afford the transplant of a heart or lung.

The intrinsic merits of many of the other principles are harder to judge. Should American citizens be a favored group in distributing organs for transplantation? Kilner suggests a 10 percent quota for nonresidents, trying to split the difference between citizens and noncitizens without suggesting any clear principle for doing so. (The figure now in effect in the transplant world is 5 percent.) And what of the practice common to transplant teams of putting patients who are about to die at the top of the list, even if they are the last to request help? Is it fair that the very sick, who may have been waiting for months, are made to wait still longer until their condition deteriorates and they are pushed to the top?

Kilner would give precedence to those facing imminent death and to those who use less of a scarce resource than others, so as to increase the number who can be treated. For example, a patient who needs dialysis once a week would take precedence over a patient who needs to be on a machine around the clock. He would also give precedence to those with "special responsibilities," that is, physicians, scientists, politicians, business leaders, and parents with dependents, who were indispensable to their family or community. Although Kilner wants a committee to screen each application and make decisions case by case, we never learn who would appoint such a committee, what would be the source of its legal or moral authority, or how it would devise criteria that were as fair to a parent of young children as to a potential Nobel laureate. By giving preference to people with "special responsibilities," Kilner revives the use of social criteria in medical decisions, with all its problems and biases.

Paul Menzel writes that "strong medicine does not always need to wait for people to sign on some dotted line to legitimize a cautious but courageous rationing of care," particularly when obtaining the explicit consent of patients would be "impossible or prohibitively costly." Instead, he assumes that individual patients have given consent to a rationing scheme if there is a strong social consensus that the action is legitimate. He takes as an example the practices of the British National Health Service in treating kidney disease. Having decided that dialysis brings only small benefits to patients over sixty-five, the British health authorities have restricted investment in dialysis centers and machines. British physicians simply inform elderly patients who need dialysis that nothing can be done for them. Menzel seems troubled that British doctors disguise the true reasons for the decision not to give treatment. He doggedly insists that such rationing has the patient's prior consent. As a voter, he argues, the patient probably supported the government's policy—at least before his kidneys failed—and in any case he or she supports the British system of parliamentary and cabinet government by which those decisions are made.

The doctor therefore not only should accept that prior consent has somehow been given but be obliged to respect it. Would the doctor "not be insulting him as an average British citizen proud of his NHS if she ignored scarcity criteria and got him on dialysis?" But why do doctors have to conceal the true situation if such a degree of prior agreement actually exists? The fact is that dissatisfaction with the health service has been growing in England, but quite aside from this Menzel has no reason for taking "prior consent" for granted in particular cases.

Menzel's closing chapter, entitled "The Duty to Die Cheaply," carries the principle of prior consent further. To forgo the use of scarce and expensive medical resources when one is terminally ill is not merely noble or heroic; "allowing oneself to die to save resources," he writes, "can indeed be one's moral duty," a duty that he believes is socially enforceable—governments may force people to die cheaply. Menzel draws on the language of Christian ethics in defending this proposition. Not to die cheaply is to pursue "our own vanity," to make "idols out of ourselves," to elevate egoism over communal obligations, and to reject the sovereignty of God over us. Fully persuaded of this, he tries to establish a connection between terminal illness and what he calls "quasi-terminal care"—treatments that will have limited benefits for people likely to die soon anyway. Since dialysis gives patients over sixty-five only a few more years of life, years that are going to be difficult and sometimes painful, in their case treatment should be withheld. Such care should also be withheld from patients who are "severely demented":

> Like low-benefit terminal care, life-extending care of the severely demented becomes a first-order candidate for restrictions if we take seriously the task of matching rationing policies with people's actual values.

Why does Menzel believe that such policies would be widely acceptable? A "significant number" of patients themselves reject dialysis, he writes, and as for those with severe dementia, the conclusion is "virtually unquestionable."

Menzel insists that "prior consent does not give a simple green light to any and all efficient policies," but he never explains when the kind of utilitarian decision-making he evidently admires should be restricted. Since he presumes, on no evidence from real life, that the consensus he believes exists will always be fairly applied, he never even considers the possibility that minorities may need protection against majorities. He is willing to deny severely demented people treatment without pondering the implications of such a policy for the severely retarded or the chronic schizophrenic.[8]

The most ambitious argument for rationing comes from Daniel Callahan. His first book on rationing medicine, *Setting Limits*,[9] addressed the narrower question of how much health care the aged should have. In *What Kind of Life* he takes up the question of how much health care Americans should be entitled to have.

Callahan contends that individual demand for health care is virtually boundless. People will pursue every technological fix to ward off disease and death, no matter how scarce or expensive. He repeatedly blames "liberal society" for not curbing "individual desires and needs," but he provides no data to back up the claim that patients' "needs, endless needs" bear the main responsibility for increasing the amount of medical treatment rather than, say, the policies of hospitals or the

---

8. I do not want to leave the impression that bioethicists are all in agreement about rationing. Samuel Gorovitz's account of the seven weeks he spent at Boston's Beth Israel Hospital (*Drawing the Line*, Oxford University Press, 1991) includes a passing reference to rationing that underlines the problems raised by Menzel's approach. Gorovitz notes that addressing questions about how to ration can become a "destructive" exercise, "for to answer them at all, even on the most tentative basis, is to devalue entire categories of people." He concedes that in the future we might be compelled to address these questions, but "until we are unable to avoid them, it may be best to keep on trying."

9. *Setting Limits: Medical Goals in an Aging Society* (Simon and Schuster, 1987).

attitude of physicians. According to Callahan, we have forgotten that medical treatments are not an end but a means to an end—health should be restored not so that we will be healthy but so that we can fulfill other goals, social, intellectual, and personal. Failure to recognize this principle undercuts our ability to set limits on treatment at a time when mounting medical costs are swallowing up resources needed to meet other pressing social needs.

Making health care more efficient, or devising new formulas to contain the costs of hospitals and physicians, or more accurately assessing medical technology will not, Callahan believes, resolve our predicament. Since, in his view, the force inexorably driving up medical costs is personal demand for more and more treatment, none of these measures would curb it. The only solution is to impose limits on how much treatment a person will get. We should provide only as much health care as is necessary to maintain in good working order the political and legal system, the national defense, the pursuit of knowledge and culture, and the institutions, ranging from the family to philanthropic organizations, that hold society together. Rather than underwrite more medical research to produce more high-technology medicine, we should be investing in schools, industrial development, highways, parks, and recreation. After all, some exceptions aside, the

> average level of individual and societal health is *already* adequate to meet the general needs.... Whatever the shortcomings of our social institutions, the poor health of their participants is not the cause.

And of the failings of American corporations, Callahan asks: "Has anyone seriously suggested that poor health is the reason we no longer compete well with the Japanese?"

When it comes to the goals of medicine, Callahan would give

precedence to care and prevention, not cure. Programs should serve first the chronic patient who requires social services (hospice, nursing, and institutional care), not the acutely ill patient who needs high-technology diagnosis or treatment. He also emphasizes the value of preventive medicine and prenatal care, along with low-tech, low-cost, and effective measures, such as providing antibiotics and simple emergency medicine. These procedures address the "common threat to all," and ensure the "adequate functioning of societal institutions." What would Callahan eliminate? He would discourage treatment of infants weighing less than five hundred grams, as well as dialysis, organ transplants, and artificial feeding and resuscitation of the elderly. Nor would he prescribe AZT for persons with AIDS. Callahan claims these expensive treatments merely solve "individualized problems" and yield a low quality of life for the patient and within the society as a whole.

Even if we grant that Callahan is right that billions of dollars are squandered in futile attempts to ward off death, the guidelines he suggests are grossly inadequate. Take his central principle: provide only that health care which the community requires to achieve stability and maintain order. In his earlier book, *Setting Limits*, he had a different argument. There he contended that the values people held were distracted by "modernism," the "belief that human ingenuity can bring about a better future...that nature is not fixed or normative in its ends but is malleable to human purposes and construction." From this premise, he put forward a concept of a "natural life span"— when one's possibilities in life have been realized—to indicate the moment when medicine "should be used not for the further extension of the life of the aged." As some critics have pointed out, Callahan confused the "natural" with the ethically desirable, and attempted to impose a seemingly objective standard (a natural life span) onto an inevitably subjective judgment (a full and satisfying life). In *What Kind of Life*, Callahan speaks not of nature but of society, yet his notion of good social order is no more persuasive as a basis for rationing medicine than is the notion of "nature."

In any case, Callahan's assumption of a clear relation between health and social stability hardly seems warranted. No one has even shown that the many defects of American social institutions since the eighteenth century were caused by the poor health of our citizens. Even in developing countries where the case for preventive medicine is obvious, Callahan's standard is of no help. In some of these countries—India is a good example—poor health is endemic and so is social disorder, but the two are not evidently related. In fact, in the name of good order, these countries prefer to devote almost all social resources to economic development, hoping that health care will improve as a byproduct of economic growth.

In the closing pages of *Setting Limits*, Callahan suddenly informs the reader that everything he has said about rationing health care and restricting individual choice applies only to public programs. If people can pay for advanced technology and medical treatment directly or through private insurance, they can have all they want no matter how old they are. Thus Callahan's elaborate arguments come down to a scheme legitimizing inequalities in health care based on wealth.

Conceding that his plan is "not too different from the system we now have in a crude form," Callahan offers one central defense of it: by no longer paying for high-tech medicine such as kidney dialysis, the government would be able to extend insurance coverage to all Americans. The two-tier medical system he proposes would finally bring us national health insurance. But would the elderly and the poor, and their advocates, be content with so limited a range of treatment? Yes, says Callahan, if they understood that health care is not an end in itself, if they recognized the communitarian ideals that he, Callahan, believes in, and if they appreciated the need to contain costs. These principles would be able "to overcome the animus of many egalitarians against anything other than one-tier medicine."

What Kind of Life is finally about what kind of life the poorer part of the population will have to accept. Callahan's vision of good order is aimed at keeping the have-nots in their place, content with 1950s medicine, while the haves enjoy twenty-first-century medicine.

Unlike the bioethicists, most medical doctors writing about rationing base their suggestions on the traditional principle that each patient, however old or poor, should get the treatment he or she needs, whatever the cost. In a forum in the *New England Journal of Medicine*, Arnold Relman, its former editor, and the late Norman Levinsky, who was a Boston University doctor, insisted that if the billions expended in the US for health care were spent sensibly, rationing would be unnecessary.[10] Relman contended that if technology were properly evaluated and used only when "medically indicated," costs would be controlled. He believed that much treatment is not really necessary (do US patients actually require three times as much open-heart surgery as Canadian patients?) and that too many expensive tests were being made (do American hospitals truly need eight times as many imaging machines as Canadian hospitals?). "All the evidence suggests," he found, "that there are vast savings to be made through the elimination of unnecessary services and facilities." Certainly Relman's charges deserve intensive inquiry to determine just how frequent the excesses he writes about are and what could be done to avoid them.

Levinsky also was "not persuaded that explicit rationing is necessary in the United States at this time." He was confident that eventually medical research will somehow find reasonably priced ways to cure disease and improve quality of life. To support the claim, he noted that the cost of preventing and treating smallpox had been eliminated and that tuberculosis sanitariums had closed. Whatever the limitations of

---

10. "Is Rationing Inevitable?," *New England Journal of Medicine*, Vol. 322 (June 21, 1990), pp. 1808–1816.

his argument—neither smallpox nor tuberculosis is a useful example for calculating the future costs of chronic disease in the elderly—Levinsky found the alternative, to sanction "the ethos of death as a communal act," unacceptable in "the wealthiest country in history."

Both writers would like to see the medical profession itself lead the country out of the morass that it helped create in the first place. Just who in the profession could or should provide such leadership they did not say. Nor did they acknowledge as strongly as they might have that many people, with some reason, see doctors as egotistical, high-handed people who are too concerned with collecting fees and insufficiently sensitive to the needs of patients. It seems highly unlikely that physicians will be granted the discretionary authority to set policy on which tests and which treatment will be withheld, as Relman and Levinsky recommended.

One of the more determined efforts by a physician to establish guidelines for medical ethics is Troyen Brennan's *Just Doctoring*.[11] Unlike many of his colleagues, he concedes the need for rationing, writing that "there must be limits on the resources that we as a society put into health care." Yet he does not want physicians unilaterally deciding which lives should be saved and which should not. Rather: "Physician decisions must be made within guidelines developed by a broad social consensus," and they should help "cost controls work in the best possible manner."

Unfortunately, Brennan says little about how that social consensus might be achieved. He does not want doctors to mislead patients as British doctors frequently do. Unlike Callahan, he does not want rationing to be arbitrary—not all eighty-year-olds are alike. Nor should rationing be uneven in its social effects—no one should be allowed to have special treatment because he is rich. He rightly worries that ability to pay will become the dominant principle and that "the poor

---

11. *Just Doctoring: Medical Ethics in the Liberal State* (University of California Press, 1991).

will likely bear the brunt of rationing." He hopes that physicians will somehow be able to prevent inequality in rationing, but Oregon's well-publicized venture provides an example of just how tenuous such expectations can be.

In July 1989, at the urging of Dr. John Kitzhaber, then president of the Oregon Senate and a former emergency room physician, the state legislature enacted a Basic Health Services Act that would expand the number of people eligible for Medicaid coverage but limit the benefits they might receive in order to keep state expenditures in line. The precipitating event was a request from the family of Coby Howard, a seven-year-old suffering from leukemia, that he be given a bone marrow transplant; the state's Medicaid program, however, did not cover transplants and the request was refused. Howard died before private collections could raise the necessary funds. The episode, as would be expected, provoked a good deal of media commentary and review of state policies. One legislator moved that transplants be covered by Oregon's Medicaid policy. Kitzhaber objected on the grounds that such a provision would benefit only a few. The better course would be to enlarge insurance coverage for all and set out the right package of benefits.

A state health services commission, dominated by health professionals, was then asked to rank all medical services by their importance, taking into account criteria such as "public values," "relative costs, benefits," and the quality of life after treatment. According to the plan, an actuarial group was then to calculate the cost of each service, and the legislature would make a lump sum appropriation. Each person receiving Medicaid would be eligible to receive a group of benefits that went as far down the list of services as the state appropriation would allow.[12]

---

12. Daniel M. Fox and Howard M. Leichter, "Rationing Care in Oregon: The New Accountability," and Lawrence D. Brown, "The National Politics of Oregon's Rationing Plan," *Health Affairs* (Summer 1991), pp. 7–51.

After one false start, in which treatment for thumb sucking and lower back pain far outranked operations for appendicitis, the health services commission devised a three-tier system—"Essential Services," "Very Important Services," and "Services Valuable to Certain Individuals"—and then ranked treatments within each category. The most important of the essential services were treatments for acute and fatal conditions which promised full recovery (repair of open neck wounds, treatment for coronary blockages). They also included maternal care, preventive care for children, contraceptive services, comfort care, and preventive services for adults. The very important services ranged from the treatment of acute and nonfatal conditions (filling dental cavities) to chronic nonfatal diseases (sinusitis, migraine headaches, psoriasis). The bottom tier included services that would help people to recover from acute and nonfatal conditions (diaper rash, conjunctivitis), infertility services (in vitro fertilization), and, finally, treatments which had minimal or no proven ability to improve the "quality of well-being" (therapies for viral warts).[13]

Editorial writers throughout the country initially hailed Oregon's plan. It was thought to be doing something admirable by taking the thousands of dollars that would otherwise bring doubtful benefits to a handful of patients (such as in vitro fertilization) and allocating that money to programs certain to promote the welfare of large groups (like prenatal care). Daniel Callahan predictably considered it a "bold and integrated" plan and Troyen Brennan found it "rational." Since the rankings of medical services were the subject of public discussion, the consensus was said to be democratically achieved. Because coverage would be extended to over 100,000 people lacking insurance, the program was said to be equitable.

But the Oregon venture makes apparent how treacherous the

---

13. Charles J. Dougherty, "Setting Health Care Priorities: Oregon's Next Steps," *Hastings Center Report*, Vol. 21 (May–June 1991), conference report, pp. 1–10.

politics of rationing are. The plan affects only the Medicaid population—therefore, only the poor bear the burden of the cutbacks and
they, in reality, subsidize the extension of medical coverage to other
poor people. Moreover, the plan does not affect the entire Medicaid
population: it exempts all services, social and medical, for the elderly,
which amount to well over half the Medicaid budget. The officials
who presented the plan said that social services are too difficult to
rank; more likely, nursing home operators and the elderly are constituencies too powerful for the legislature to penalize. Nor did Oregon extend its policy to the state insurance program that covers its
own employees, and it specifically prohibited any cutbacks in payment for hospitals and physicians. Thus, the one target is low-income
women and their children. Oregon's Basic Health Services Act seems
less a brave adventure than the kind of rationing limited to recipients
of public aid envisioned by Callahan.

The subsequent history of the plan is even more instructive. Three
well-known political scientists, Jonathan Oberlander, Theodore
Marmor, and Lawrence Jacobs, followed up the initiative and found
that, first, there was actually no rationing of services in Oregon.[14]
The number of services excluded from the roster, those below the line
of funding, was relatively small and unimportant. Oregon's Medicaid
plan is actually more generous than most other states. Second, physicians have become quite adept at gaming the system. They will find a
category that fits above the line even if the real diagnosis would not
get Medicaid approval. (The fine art of gaming goes on in the context
of health maintenance organizations' coverage and Medicare coverage as well. It may only be a matter of time before it becomes a medical school course.) Third, the program has not saved Oregon any

---

14. Jonathan Oberlander, Theodore Marmor, and Lawrence Jacobs, "Rationing Medical
Care: Rhetoric and Reality in the Oregon Health Plan," *Canadian Medical Association Journal*, Vol. 164 (May 29, 2001), pp. 1583–1587.

significant money; estimates are that the new system brought a 2 percent saving over the old system. Given the relatively few services that were excluded and the physicians' ability to game, this result is not surprising. Finally, Oregon has not served as a model for other states. No one else has duplicated its effort. So in sum, the worst fears about the Oregon plan have not been realized; the poor were not victimized even though they were singled out. At the same time, the ostensible benefits of rationing have not been realized either.

In view of such deep prejudices against making available to the poor the medical treatment most people would want, are we left to choose between inequity and insolvency? There is little reason for optimism in a society where indifference toward the less well-off is taken for granted; but some changes in perception may be taking place. The apocalyptic literature on rationing presupposes an insatiable demand of individual patients for high-tech medicine. But if such books as Philip Roth's *Patrimony*[15] and Andrew Malcolm's *Someday*[16] are any sign, middle-class consumers of medical care may have become more willing to accept limits on how much can be done. This reflects not a recognition of a duty to die cheaply but an unwillingness to prolong the dying process needlessly. There may now be fewer guilt-ridden families who insist that their parents spend their last days miserably in an intensive-care unit at a cost of $50,000 or more.

Roth and Malcolm describe how they decided that "everything" should not be done to postpone the inevitable. Herman Roth, the author's eighty-six-year-old father, had a non-malignant tumor pressing against the brain stem that could have been excised by surgery. Although the operation has a 75 percent survival rate (and undoubtedly would have been paid for by Medicare), it requires, depending

---

15. *Patrimony: A True Story* (Simon and Schuster, 1991).

16. Knopf, 1991.

on which surgeon you talk to, either one eight- to ten-hour operation or two seven- to eight-hour operations several months apart; the recovery period takes another several months, and Mr. Roth would have to learn how to walk again. The surgeons who saw him were certainly ready to do the operation, and they were confident Herman Roth would be worse off if he didn't have it—a standard argument of surgeons eager to perform debatable operations. But Herman Roth, with his family's agreement, did not want it. The son had his father sign a living will, refusing "mechanical respiration when I am no longer able to sustain my own breathing." Yet the end was a trial:

> Early on the morning of his death, when I arrived at the hospital emergency room ... I was confronted by an attending physician prepared to take "extraordinary measures" and to put him on a breathing machine. Without it there was no hope, though, needless to say—the doctor added—the machine wasn't going to reverse the progress of the tumor.... And I, who had explained to my father the provisions of the living will and got him to sign it, didn't know what to do.... How could I take it on myself to decide that my father should be finished with life, life which is ours to know just once? Far from invoking the living will, I was nearly on the verge of ignoring it and saying, "Anything! Anything!"

Andrew Malcolm, whose mother was suffering from lung cancer, had much the same experience, and he and Roth use almost the same language when they describe the decision to "let" their parents "go." The choice they made is becoming more frequent all the time. It has nothing to do with budgets or with concern for the commonweal, but with a recognition of futility, a desire to prevent pain, and an acceptance of the inevitable. Still, since 10 percent of health care dollars are now spent on elderly people in their last year of life, considerable savings would result if many more people made similar decisions.

Although advanced directives and proxy consent forms are still not as common as one might like, despite the fact that hospitals are required to ask, and do ask, every incoming patient whether he or she has such a document, more and more people are finding medical intervention less acceptable than a quiet death. The choices patients make consistent with this lesson will not provide a comprehensive solution to allocating resources for health care. Nor will they break the deadlock over national health insurance. Still, it seems preferable, at least for now, to rely upon modest hopes to curtail expenditures and to try to make access to medicine more democratic. The discrimination that the poor suffer in health care should not become the excuse for putting into effect clumsy and ill-conceived rationing schemes. Their consequences may well turn out to be at least as grievous as the inequalities they aim to resolve.

6

THE RIGHT TO HEALTH CARE:
LESSONS FROM SOUTH AFRICA

IN 1997, a forty-one-year-old unemployed resident of Durban, South Africa, invoked one of the most extraordinary provisions of South Africa's new constitution in a desperate court battle to save his life. Thiagraj Soobramoney was a very sick man, suffering from kidney failure along with diabetes, cardiac disease, and vascular disease, which had recently brought on a stroke. Until 1997, Soobramoney had been able to pay for his three dialysis sessions per week at a local private hospital. But then he ran out of money and when his debt to the hospital reached $25,000, the facility refused to continue his treatment. Soobramoney immediately asked one of Durban's public hospitals, Aberdeen, if he could go on one of its machines. Aberdeen said no, explaining that he did not meet its criteria for treatment. With only twenty machines and a limited staff and budget, it restricted dialysis to those about to receive a kidney transplant and to acutely ill patients who with the help of the procedure might be expected to recover, which meant excluding those with chronic conditions who probably would not. Soobramoney's multiple medical problems made him ineligible for free dialysis.

The South African constitution, which took effect in 1994, includes a number of social and economic rights not found in the US Constitution, including the rights of access to health care, housing, food, water, social security, and education. Its drafters hoped that such provisions would benefit those who had suffered under apartheid, many of whom remained poor and vulnerable. The constitutional clauses that Soobramoney cited in his court case appeared to establish his right to treatment: "Everyone has the right to have access to health care.... No one may be refused emergency medical treatment.... Everyone has the right to life." If these provisions applied to anyone, surely it was Soobramoney. Without dialysis, he would die. He first went to the lower court in Durban, which ruled against him. He then appealed to South Africa's highest court, its Constitutional Court, which also rejected his plea. Within a week of its decision, Soobramoney was dead, an event widely covered in the South African press. Arthur Chaskalson, the Constitutional Court judge who wrote the opinion denying treatment to Soobramoney, received a number of angry and abusive letters.

Why did Chaskalson and his colleagues turn Soobramoney down? It was not for lack of sensitivity to the great income disparities in South Africa. As the court noted, "Many do not have access to clean water or to adequate health services." Recognizing that these problems predated the constitution, the court wrote that "our new constitutional order" is committed "to transform our society into one in which there will be human dignity, freedom and equality." But it went on to explain that South Africa confronted daunting social and economic challenges, which the constitution also took into account: the clause immediately following the sentences on health rights declared that "the state must take reasonable legislative and other measures, within its available resources." The enforcement of those rights, in other words, is limited by the resources at the state's disposal. Confronting widespread deprivation, the state has to make choices, and so do hospitals, even if the choices are agonizing and require giving preference to the acutely ill over the chronically ill. If dialysis were given to all patients who required it, the court reasoned—indeed, if advanced medical technologies were made available to all who would benefit from them—the health care budget would overwhelm all of the state's other financial needs.

Soobramoney v. *Minister of Health* was the first decision reached by the South African Constitutional Court on social and economic rights. It framed the approach the court has taken in other cases involving such rights, including the right to housing and, most recently, the right to medical treatment to prevent the transmission of HIV from mothers to newborns. In each decision, the court struck a different balance, but its opinions demonstrated how a constitutional commitment to such rights can also accommodate practical consider-ations. This was a genuine achievement for South African jurispru-dence, and it is relevant to similar debates beyond South Africa's borders. The court's thoughtful reasoning helps to cut through the ongoing controversy around the world about the wisdom of codify-ing some types of universal rights, such as the right to health, that may or may not be enforceable.

A few years after the Soobramoney case, the Constitutional Court returned to the question of economic and social rights in *Province of Western Cape* v. *Grootboom*. In this instance, it faced the question of whether the right to housing was also limited by resources available to the state.

Irene Grootboom was one of 390 adults and 510 children who were evicted in 1999 from their squatter settlement in Oostenberg, a township on the outskirts of Cape Town. They had moved to Oosten-berg a year earlier to escape even more intolerable conditions in a nearby town, where they lacked not only water, sewage, refuse removal, and electricity but also had to endure the effects of winter floods. Despite these past hardships, the Oostenberg municipal gov-ernment only wanted to be rid of them. In an action reminiscent of apartheid days, the city bulldozed their huts and trashed their personal possessions. The desperate squatters then moved onto a sports field in the town, but when the winter rains arrived, the plastic sheets with which they wrapped their shacks gave no protection. They were back in the same hellish conditions.

Their plight came to the attention of the Legal Resources Centre in Cape Town, a public interest law firm funded for many years by the Ford Foundation. Its lawyers sued first in the Cape of Good Hope High Court, and won limited relief. The court ruled that children and one of their parents had to be provided with some form of housing; all others were to receive tents, toilets, and a regular supply of trucked-in water. The government appealed this ruling to the Constitutional Court.

In its opinion, issued in October 2000, the Constitutional Court began by observing that the desperate housing shortages in South Africa were rooted in apartheid, and particularly in the white government's determination to exclude Africans from urban areas. The court then turned to the first clause in Section 26 of the constitution, which states that "everyone has a right to have access to adequate housing," and addressed the question of whether the court could order the state to fulfill such a right. Should the court be making decisions about the budget and the allocation of resources, or should that be left to the executive and legislative branches?

The court had no reservations on how to answer the general question: social and economic rights were indeed subject to judicial review and intervention. The constitution obliges the state "to respect, protect, promote, and fulfill such rights," and the court must insure that those obligations are met. The court's responsibility was not only to prevent the state from interfering with these rights but also to ensure that they were effectively enforced. How was the court to fulfill this charge? As they did in *Soobramoney*, the justices did not impose a single formula, preferring instead to weigh competing claims. Pragmatism had to be joined to principle, an approach that the court argued was intrinsic to the letter and spirit of the South African constitution.

In *Grootboom*, the court was again guided by the constitutional clause that followed the statement of housing rights, specifying that "the state must take reasonable legislative and other measures, within its available resources, to achieve the progressive realisation of this right." To satisfy these provisions, the court wrote, the state had to devise a "workable" housing plan, not necessarily an ideal but a "reasonable" one. A policy that discriminated against a "significant sector of society" or a policy that ignored people with the most pressing and urgent needs would not pass the test. However, a policy that took into account resource constraints and set down a timetable for eventual rather than immediate implementation would meet it.

The court went to some trouble to differentiate the South African mandates from the provisions embodied in universal declarations. The 1966 International Covenant on Economic, Social, and Cultural Rights, for example, proclaims a right to adequate housing; the South African provision, however, provides "a right to access to adequate housing." The International Covenant charges governments to take "appropriate steps" to secure the right. In South Africa, the state must take "reasonable" measures.

In the case of Irene Grootboom and her fellow squatters, the court found that the municipality's plan for their housing was inadequate, and it condemned their callous treatment. But it rejected the plaintiffs' call for "immediate relief," ruling that a remedy needed to be "timely." (We were told that the court considered invoking the idea of "all deliberate speed," but decided to avoid the controversy that has raged around the US Supreme Court's use of the phrase in *Brown* v. *Board of Education*, its 1954 decision that segregated schools were unconstitutional.) The court did not prescribe a housing plan; rather, it ordered the municipality to devise one that met the plaintiffs' needs and to carry it out in such a way that there would be "an end in sight." In effect, it had to be reasonable.

* * *

The third case in which the Constitutional Court addressed social and economic rights was *Minister of Health* v. *Treatment Action Campaign*. Decided in July 2002, the case examined whether the state was obligated to supply HIV-positive mothers with the drug nevirapine to prevent transmission of the virus to their newborns.[1] Although nevirapine's efficacy had been well established, the South African government, following the lead of its president, Thabo Mbeki, was unwilling to distribute it widely. It claimed the drug's safety was still in question. It also maintained that because breast feeding by HIV-positive mothers might still transmit the virus, it had to consider providing formula milk. So instead of making nevirapine easily and immediately available to all, the government wanted to restrict the drug to two pilot research sites in each province for a period of two years. These pilot programs would allow time for, among other things, improved management and "community mobilization efforts."

An unusual coalition of advocates, physicians, and lawyers opposed the government plan. The primary organizer was the Treatment Action Campaign (TAC), formed in 1998 and spearheaded by Zachie Achmat, an openly gay AIDS activist who had previously been a fierce agitator against apartheid. TAC's main goal was to force the South African government to adopt an effective treatment program for AIDS and to shame pharmaceutical companies into reducing prices of antiretroviral drugs. The group organized protest marches, carried out campaigns in the press, and eventually took the government to court. In addition, a Johannesburg pediatrician, Haroon Saloojee, organized Save Our Babies, a group that advised TAC on medical matters and encouraged other doctors to join the protest. From the coalition's standpoint, making nevirapine widely available was not only vital in

---

1. The ethics of the research establishing the efficacy of AZT and nevirapine is discussed in Chapter 3, "The Shame of Medical Research."

itself but was also an excellent starting point for a more general campaign to make retroviral treatment available for all persons with AIDS.[2]

Over 1999 and 2000, TAC continued to organize demonstrations, petition the government, and negotiate with the Ministry of Health over nevirapine. Its efforts, however, brought no changes. Its frustrations were compounded by President Mbeki's open support for so-called "AIDS dissidents," a small group of scientists who questioned both the severity of the epidemic and the viral causes of HIV/AIDS, and by his insistence that antiretroviral drugs were poisons. Then in April 2001, the TAC campaign won an important victory: the Medicines Control Council (MCC), the South African equivalent of the US Food and Drug Administration, approved the use of nevirapine against mother-to-child transmission, judging it safe and effective. When even that finding did not affect government policy, TAC filed a lawsuit demanding that the government distribute the drug free to pregnant women in all public hospitals. In December, the Pretoria High Court decided in favor of TAC, whereupon the government appealed to the Constitutional Court.

The court upheld the Pretoria ruling, with Justice Arthur Chaskalson again writing the opinion. The government, he noted, offered three justifications: the drug was not yet proven safe and effective; the issues raised by TAC could not be decided by the courts because social and economic issues belonged to the executive and legislative branches of government; and the Ministry of Health needed more time to assess the "operational challenges" of distributing the drug.

The court dismissed the first point because every health organization, from the World Health Organization to the South African MCC,

---

2. This account draws on our interview with Mark Heywood in January 2003 and his article "Preventing Mother-to-Child HIV Transmission in South Africa: Background Strategies and Outcomes of the Treatment Action Campaign Case Against the Minister of Health," *South African Journal of Human Rights*, Vol. 19 (2003), pp. 278–315.

had found that the benefits of nevirapine outweighed its risks. Indeed, as the court observed, private hospitals in South Africa were dispensing it to all HIV-positive expectant mothers. As to the court's jurisdiction, the question "is not whether socio-economic rights are justiciable. Clearly, they are." The core issue was whether, in light of a constitutional right to access to health care, the state's policy was reasonable, timely, and proportionate to its available resources.

The Chaskalson opinion found that the state's policy met none of these requirements. The very ease with which nevirapine could be dispensed distinguished it from dialysis: all that was required was a single dose administered to mothers immediately before delivery and to newborns shortly thereafter. The drug was inexpensive, and its manufacturer, Boehringer, had offered to provide it for five years without cost. Moreover, some public clinics were already dispensing it successfully. In Capetown, the deputy director of health, Faried Abdullah, was providing nevirapine to practically all HIV-positive women and their newborns.

Thus, the court concluded, the government plan violated basic constitutional rights. In the *Grootboom* housing case, the court had condemned "a program that excludes a significant segment of society," and this was precisely the effect of the government's nevirapine policy. Those who could afford private care were well served; patients in the public health system had to suffer from the transmission of a deadly disease. The court's responsibility was to prevent the government from creating obstacles to the fulfillment of social and economic rights and, further, to compel it to carry out programs to realize these rights. Accordingly, the court ordered the government to end all restrictions on nevirapine in public hospitals and to make it widely available for physician use.

What impact have the court's rulings had on the conduct of public policy? Has its skillful balancing of pragmatic and principled considerations advanced social and economic rights? Put another way, when the court speaks, does anyone in South Africa listen?

The answer is yes, but only to a point. Because of the *Grootboom* decision, the government added special provisions for emergency relief to its housing plans. And since *Grootboom*, the court has returned several more times to the issue, pressing the government to meet the needs of its most desperate citizens and supporting its efforts to do so. At the end of the summer of 2000, heavy rains flooded parts of Alexandra Township on the outskirts of Johannesburg, uprooting some three hundred families. The government arranged a temporary settlement for them on nearby state-owned land, whereupon those living in neighboring Kyalami objected and went to court. Their central argument was that the government action violated their property rights because the new settlement would drive down the value of their land and homes. The case made its way to the Constitutional Court, which ruled in favor of the state. Although it recognized that a conflict of rights was involved, it gave primacy to the interests of the flood victims: they had to be allowed to remain where they were. In effect, as some critics were quick to note, it elevated socioeconomic rights above property rights.

But when no emergency existed and alternatives were available, the court ordered the government both to respect property rights and provide access to housing. In May 2000, after some two thousand people illegally occupied land on a privately owned farm, Modderklip, on the outskirts of Johannesburg, the owners tried to get the government first to purchase the property, and when that failed, to evict the settlers, whose numbers eventually grew to 40,000. When the government refused to do anything at all, the company that owned the property filed suit. In May 2005, the Constitutional Court ruled in favor of the property owners: "It is unreasonable for a private entity such as Modderklip to be forced to bear the burden which should be borne by the state of providing occupiers with accommodation."

According to the Court, such occupations "have the potential to have serious implications for stability and public peace." If the state does not protect private property, it is "a recipe for anarchy." It then ordered the government to compensate the company for the land occupied since May 2000 and also ruled that the settlers could remain there until other land was made available. In February 2006, the government declared that moving the residents, who by now numbered 70,000, to another site was a "priority," and would occur "shortly." But no date was set for the relocation.

Lower courts have followed the approach set down in *Grootboom*, insisting that the government meet its constitutional responsibilities in "timely" fashion. In this spirit, the High Court of Cape Town in 2003 ordered the city to provide housing for some eighty squatters on public land in the township of Valhalla Park who were in a "desperate situation." Some of them had been on municipal waiting lists for housing for ten years, and were living in shacks, abandoned buildings, backyards, or on the streets; two of them were living out of cars. The municipality dallied, denying that the claimants were in emergency conditions and claiming that other people needed housing too; the court kept prodding it to give short-term relief even as it planned for the longer term. In December 2005, the court found that at long last the city had acknowledged its responsibility for alleviating the situation, that it had agreed not to evict the Valhalla Park settlers, and that the emergency conditions had been mitigated. It might have issued what is known in South African law as a "structural interdict," ordering the city to act immediately and report back regularly on its progress. But it refrained, finding that the city was now behaving in a responsible fashion. It was probably also trying to avoid a direct confrontation between the judicial branch and the executive branch of government.

In effect, because a right to access to housing is embedded in the South African constitution, the Constitutional Court has become a participant in the allocation of scarce public resources. Even a government in what is essentially a one-party state will be reluctant to be condemned by its own justices. The court has exercised its authority very carefully, recognizing the complexity of enforcing rights in a society with a legacy of apartheid and limited resources. Critics of the court are impatient with what they consider to be its timidity and its reluctance to order the government to take immediate remedial action. After all, some two million households still live in "informal housing structures," that is, in shacks on public or private land or in rooms inside abandoned buildings or houses. But the court clearly prefers to negotiate rather than to command, to urge the state to meet its constitutional responsibilities, and not to make itself responsible for implementing them.

The Constitutional Court's ruling that the state must make nevirapine available for public use has also confronted a series of barriers, different but no less challenging that those in housing. No one in the South African government opposes the principle of providing adequate housing, but many of them do share an uncompromising hostility toward providing drugs to combat AIDS.

The Mbeki government at first appeared to accept the nevirapine judgment. A spokesperson for the Ministry of Health found it "workable." TAC, for its part, postponed a scheduled civil disobedience action and announced its readiness to negotiate with the government and to assist with implementing a treatment program. But the truce quickly dissolved and acrimony continued. In August 2002, one month after the court's decision, the MCC declared that it was reviewing its approval of nevirapine, citing the fact that the FDA was examining the clinical trial of the drug carried out in Uganda. Because the FDA was concerned less with the efficacy of the drug and more with the procedures followed in the clinical trial, it seemed obvious to TAC that the MCC was caving in to government pressures to reverse its earlier approval.

Eventually, the MCC backed off, and the use of nevirapine increased, albeit unevenly. Where a provincial government was steadfastly loyal to Mbeki, as was true in Mpumalanga, a province about an hour north of Johannesburg, the drug was not available. On the other hand, Johannesburg's three-thousand-bed public hospital, Baragwanath, dispensed nevirapine to everyone who needed it. So did the health facilities in the Western Cape and in Durban. Since no government office tracked the use of the drug, accurate statistics are not available, but it seems that no less than several hundred thousand mothers and their infants have benefited from it—no small achievement even in a country with five million cases of AIDS. Without the court's intervention, it is very doubtful that these numbers would have been reached.

The court decision also provided some protection to health professionals who were otherwise at the mercy of a politically ruthless government. For example, some doctors in Mpumalanga's public hospital who were unable to obtain nevirapine from the facility had paid for the drug out of their own pockets and given it to their patients. They were then dismissed, on the dubious grounds that only drugs paid for from public funds could be used in public hospitals. After the court ruling, such firings stopped.

Nevirapine soon confronted another challenge, however. As had long been known, a single dose of the drug may put the mother who receives it at risk for developing resistance to all antiretroviral compounds. In combating AIDS, as in treating tuberculosis, a single-drug therapy is not as effective as a combination of drugs. The very best regimen to follow in order to prevent mother-to-child transmission is to give the expectant mother AZT starting at twenty-eight weeks, then supplement it with nevirapine when she is about to give birth. In July 2004, when new clinical findings confirmed the superiority of this approach, the MCC recommended that all single doses of nevirapine be discontinued and that the more complicated combination therapy be instituted.

The MCC's recommendation was intended not to improve the level of health care but to stall a program the government did not want to support. Responsible medical groups within and outside of South Africa objected, noting that the government had not committed itself to distribute the more expensive AZT-nevirapine combination. Moreover, because many rural women did not go to a health clinic until childbirth was imminent, they would be unable to have access to the more complicated regimen. So few HIV-positive mothers were likely to receive combination therapy that the risk of future resistance that might come from a single dose of nevirapine was nearly irrelevant. Finally, clinical investigators were confident that only a small number of women taking the single dose of nevirapine would actually develop resistance, and it was likely to be short-term.

With good reason, TAC activists concluded that only the government's bizarre attitudes toward AIDS therapy could explain why it would want to abandon single-dose nevirapine and permit certain contagion and death. As one of them declared:

> The Minister of Health has been up to her old tricks.... She is now misreading...scientific findings that nevirapine in conjunction with AZT is better than nevirapine alone, and using this to vindicate her antagonism to nevirapine. She is basically implying that she was compelled through the courts (by TAC) to introduce a prophylactic intervention which she in her infinite wisdom knew was dangerous! And now she can say "I told you so."

Undoubtedly the parties will be back in court again, and in all likelihood the justices will rule in TAC's favor. The most recent data strongly support the efficacy and safety of nevirapine: mothers who had successfully taken the drug when delivering their first child and avoided transmission do not pass on the virus after they take it again for their second child. Treatment will be uneven and progress slow, but because of the court's defense of social and economic rights, thousands of future newborns will escape a sentence of AIDS.

An appreciation of the performance of the South African Constitutional Court can help clarify some of the arguments over the usefulness of sweeping international declarations of a right to health. The first was the Universal Declaration of Human Rights, adopted by the UN General Assembly in 1948: it proclaimed that everyone had a right to "a standard of living adequate for health and well-being," which included "medical care" as well as food, clothing, and housing. In 1966, the International Covenant on Economic, Social, and Cultural Rights set forth "the right of everyone to the enjoyment of the highest attainable standard of physical and mental health." States were obliged to reduce infant mortality, promote the healthy development of the child, prevent, treat, and control epidemics, and create the "conditions which would assure to all medical service and medical attention in the event of sickness." In its 1948 constitution, the World Health Organization said that "the enjoyment of the highest attainable standard of health is one of the fundamental rights of every human being." The 1978 Declaration of Alma-Ata, Kazakhstan, reaffirmed the WHO's position, noted the disparities between developed and underdeveloped countries, and called upon all governments to provide health and social benefits. By the year 2000, the declaration proclaimed, "all peoples of the world" should enjoy a level of health that allows for "a socially and economically productive life."

The ambitious goals of these declarations have obviously not been met. Malaria persists, as do tuberculosis and of course AIDS. Moreover, many developing countries also suffer from a continuing, even worsening, shortage of medical personnel (who often move to richer countries) as well as of drugs and health care facilities. All the while, the pollution and occupational hazards that accompany economic development take their toll on health. To be sure, some major victories have been won, such as the near eradication of polio. But a quarter-century after the Alma-Ata statement, health is still only for some, and inequities persist almost everywhere.

Although no one minimizes the difficulties of the problems that undercut a right to health, some critics have taken issue with the declarations themselves, finding them inconsistent and overblown. A human rights framework, they argue, cannot be imposed on health care or, for that matter, on other economic and social conditions. The principles of human rights, in this view, work best as limitations on governments, specifying actions that they may not undertake. Thus, human rights principles properly prohibit governments from the practice of torture and arbitrary arrest and detention. States, regardless of their economic resources, are able to abide by them. The standard for compliance is everywhere the same; adherence can be monitored and abuses can be exposed. When torture occurs, whether in Argentina, Serbia, Iraq, or Guantánamo, it will sooner or later be revealed and condemned.

By contrast, these critics insist, rights that require the provision of goods and services, such as health, rather than the prevention of a practice such as torture, cannot mean the same thing in a poor country as in a rich country. And rights that purport to be universal ought not to vary by per capita income or economic productivity. Moreover, while one can carefully define what constitutes the practice of torture, no one can know for certain what it means for a government to provide good health. It can build hospitals and train health professionals, but that may not be enough to deliver on the promise.

Finally, critics do not find these declarations helpful in guiding government priorities. Should health care always be the first appropriation to be made? A nation may decide that its people's well-being will be better advanced by building more roads and factories rather than hospitals. The situation gets even more muddied when the WHO and Alma-Ata declarations define health not only as a "mere" absence of disease but a satisfactory physical, psychological, social, and economic state. Exactly how are resource-poor nations to realize all these goals?

By contrast, the need to set forth and promote social and economic rights has staunch defenders who believe that governments should be held to standards that provide citizens with genuine dignity. If a government does not promote health, they argue, all other rights are diminished. Citizens cannot exercise their rights when they are hungry or homeless or lack access to doctors and medicines. While some diseases can strike anyone, malaria, diarrhea, malnutrition, tuberculosis, and AIDS disproportionately occur among people who are poor and vulnerable.

Proponents are also beginning to trim back the all-encompassing definitions of a right to health. In December 2005, Mary Robinson, former UN High Commissioner for Human Rights, and Paul Hunt, the United Nations Special Rapporteur on the Right to the Highest Attainable Standard of Health, issued a Right to Health statement with signatories ranging from Bono to Václav Havel. It opens by noting that a right to health is not a right to be healthy, nor does it mean that governments must fund expensive health services. What constitutes a right to health is the provision of clean water, sanitation, accountability in health care decisions, the abolition of user fees for primary health care, and training of health care workers. Although aimed at countries rich and poor, the target audience is clearly the developed world, which is being urged to give improvements in health a central place in global efforts to reduce poverty and encourage economic development.

This statement is more in tune than most of its predecessors with the lessons that may be drawn from the South African experience. Its constitution is a model for recognizing social and economic rights and its court has interpreted them in a manner that demonstrates how fundamental principles such as the right to health care or housing need not be merely grandiose phrases. Rather, when appropriately defined and interpreted, such rights can set the standards that a government must aim to satisfy. The Constitutional Court cannot enforce such rights, but its decisions can provide leverage to advocacy groups, serve to educate the public, and force a hostile or indifferent government to act in ways that help bring greater dignity, freedom, and equality to its people. As the court has so ably recognized, the force of a right to health lies not in uplifting slogans such as "health for all," but in a nation's ability to unite an idealistic sense of people's needs with a pragmatic sense of what its resources allow.

IV

Protection from Medical Harm

7

DEATH IN ZIMBABWE

THE DEATH OF one child from possible medical malpractice at a private hospital in Harare, the capital of Zimbabwe, might not seem like a case of human rights abuse on a continent where literally millions of people are dying from starvation and AIDS, and continue to suffer from such preventable diseases as cholera, dysentery, polio, and tetanus. But the difficulties encountered in Harare by Charles and Mary Khaminwa as they tried to make the medical profession accountable for the death of their daughter Lavender in August 1990 raise fundamental questions about the relations between professional responsibility and a respect for human rights. What are the consequences when medicine—or, for that matter, law, journalism, the academy, or the clergy—fails to uphold basic ethical standards against the self-interest of its members? And if the profession places no restraints on greed and health care is left unregulated in a free-market economy, who will protect citizens from the arbitrary use of authority, whether by doctors in hospitals or by guards in prisons? The events recounted below occurred over the period from 1990 to 1992, before the government of Robert Mugabe became completely corrupt and brutal. However, there are portents here of the consequences of his policies for Zimbabwe and the well-being of its citizens.

* * *

On February 12, 1991, Charles and Mary Khaminwa wrote to the Washington office of Africa Watch requesting help that would "enable us to continue our legal struggle to bring to book those responsible for the death of our child, the late Miss Lavender Muhonja Precious Khaminwa." As their letter explained, the Khaminwas were a Kenyan couple who had moved to Harare in 1984 so that Charles, a lawyer with several years' training in the US, could direct a community development project. Ten-year-old Lavender, their eldest child, had been attending a private boarding school on the outskirts of Harare. During the first week of August 1990, she came home complaining of stomach pains; when the Khaminwas took her to the family pediatrician, he recommended that she see a surgeon. "On 9 August 1990," the Khaminwas recounted, "Lavender was admitted to a local private hospital, the Avenues Clinic in Harare.... On 10th August 1990, she was subjected to an appendectomy and died suddenly a few hours later."

On the basis of autopsy reports, statements made by the physicians and nurses, and reports of other cases in Harare of death or disability from anesthesia, the Khaminwas were convinced that "Lavender was the victim of wrong, unorthodox, hazardous and seemingly experimental treatment, and of poor or non-existent post-operative and post-anesthetic surveillance and care." For six months they had tried to persuade the Zimbabwean medical societies and public officials to investigate the circumstances of her death, but had been so far unsuccessful. "We have been shocked to discover the extent to which medicine ... seems to be operating in an ethical vacuum. A deficit of control exists in the monitoring apparatus." The politicians "leave their medical communities to more or less administer themselves"; physicians inevitably cover up for each other, and average patients, whose "fear of authority, any kind of authority, had become so ingrained," cannot even imagine mounting a protest. The Khaminwas' extraordinary struggle appeared to embody a concern for health care as a basic right, and so, on behalf of Africa Watch, we went to Zimbabwe to meet them and learn more about the case.

Zimbabwe is one of the handful of African countries that left the existing economic establishment intact after it became independent. When Robert Mugabe took power in 1980, overturning the Rhodesian regime of Ian Smith after a decade of insurgency, he chose to placate the whites, hoping to avoid a flight that would deprive Zimbabwe not only of capital but also of people with managerial and technical skills. His principle of reconciliation was expressed in his motto, "I have drawn a line through the past."[1] It seemed that Zimbabwe, at least, was trying to establish a new model for the transfer of power from whites to blacks, without a reign of terror or corruption or economic decline.

Thus most Rhodesian officials who had violated human rights, former prime minster Ian Smith included, were never prosecuted, and in spite of staggering differences in wealth between whites and blacks, Mugabe, during his first decade as prime minister, did not confiscate white-owned land, including the rich and profitable tobacco farms. (In March 2005, he pushed through legislation allowing the state to forcibly acquire white-owned land at less than market value; it is still not clear whether he will exercise this authority in the face of possible challenges from the Zimbabwe Supreme Court as well as from foreign sources of aid like the International Monetary Fund and the World Bank.)

In matters of health and welfare, Mugabe's socialist regime has permitted many private services such as health and education to exist along with public ones, so that wealth has replaced race as the decisive factor in a segregated society. Expensive private schools educate mainly white children, apart from all but a few privileged blacks, and costly private physicians and private hospitals treat white patients, apart from all but the most well-off blacks.

---

1. Quoted in Richard Carver's October 1989 report for Africa Watch, "Zimbabwe: A Break with the Past?," pp. 9–10.

From the government's perspective, this two-track system has many advantages. In medicine, it keeps white discontent to a minimum, while shifting the entire financial burden for obtaining modern medical care to the white community. At the same time, public medical funds are free to be used to underwrite preventive health care programs, which have brought some genuine gains to the rural poor. During the 1980s, state expenditures for child and maternal health doubled (from 7 to 14 percent). Infant mortality declined (from 97 per 1,000 births in 1970 to 68 per 1,000 in 1990), and the number of babies fully vaccinated against whooping cough, tetanus, polio, and measles more than doubled (from 25 to between 50 and 80 percent).[2]

But in spite of these advances, blacks in Zimbabwe still receive only the most rudimentary medical services. They depend almost exclusively on village health workers who know little about and can do almost nothing for most of the common diseases that affect adults, including hypertension, diabetes, and cancer. Most of those who suffer from these diseases go untreated, and the few who do eventually get medical attention arrive at clinics in so advanced a stage that interventions are usually futile. In effect, whites have access to the latest technologies while blacks get little more than inoculations.

Moreover, the progress made in prevention is being canceled out by the spreading AIDS epidemic. Zimbabwean public health officials estimated in the early 1990s that 500,000 people out of a population of ten million were infected with the virus, a rate equal to that of Uganda; others, including the US Agency for International Development, put the number at one million and calculated that 25 to 30

---

2. Rene Loewenson, David Sanders, and Rob Davies, "Challenges to Equity in Health and Health Care: A Zimbabwean Case Study," *Social Science and Medicine*, Vol. 32 (1991), p. 1086; US Agency for International Development, Bureau for Africa, "Country Report: Zimbabwe," January 1991; see also the "Report of the [Zimbabwean] Secretary for Health for... 1981, Harare," p. 19, and the World Bank, *Sub-Sahara Africa: From Crisis to Sustainable Growth* (Washington, D.C., 1989), p. 69.

percent of those between the ages of twenty and forty years old, and 40 to 60 percent of those in the military, were HIV-positive. Although information about the AIDS epidemic is no longer censored, the problem is still not widely discussed, and, from what we could learn, most AIDS patients are simply sent home to die.[3] In any case, Mugabe's government has almost completely neglected the public hospitals. Under Rhodesian rule, there were two public hospitals in Harare. The one for whites, then called Andrew Fleming and now Parirenyatwa, was located in one of the most exclusive neighborhoods, near the university medical school; the ratios of nurses and doctors to patients and the expenditures per patient were all comparable to those of a hospital in London. The hospital for blacks, Harare Central, was nearer the black neighborhood and woefully lacking in funds. After independence, the two hospitals were racially integrated and put under the same administration, but this brought no improvement for Harare Central, while the care at the former whites-only hospital declined in quality. Now the wards of both hospitals are desperately overcrowded and understaffed, and even the most basic medical equipment is lacking.[4]

Many in the white community had expected that public health services would become worse with independence; even before Mugabe came to power whites were arranging for the construction of their own private, for-profit hospitals, among them the Avenues Clinic, where Lavender died. In the late 1970s, a number of corporations and private investors joined together to pay for its construction costs,

---

3. Jane Perlez, "Educational Effort Fights AIDS in Zimbabwe," *The New York Times*, April 12, 1992, p. 18; US Agency for International Development, Bureau for Africa, Country Profile, Zimbabwe, January 1991, p. 1.

4. An underground newspaper, *The Insider*, had as its lead story: "Inside a Hospital: Dr cries as child dies because he can't find right drug. Nurse collapses and there is no equipment to help her" (December 1991/January 1992).

and in 1981, the clinic opened, with two hundred beds ready to serve Harare's whites, and the few blacks who could afford its considerable fees.[5] The sponsors looked forward to handsome returns on their investments, and the patients to first-class medical care.

The outcome, however, has been far from a success. Avenues Clinic has clean corridors, a well-stocked pharmacy, and the newest medical technologies. But the medicine practiced there is often shoddy and the incompetence among the physicians frightening. This situation has a variety of causes, but the main problem is that no one will hold the hospitals or the staff accountable for their actions—not the state, not the investors, and not the profession itself.

Maintaining effective oversight of medicine is never easy anywhere, but the US and most other developed countries have procedures to identify negligent and incompetent physicians, and to discipline or remove them from practice. These include weekly staff meetings (known as morbidity and mortality rounds) to review the course of treatment for each patient who dies while in the hospital (did the physicians miss something and how might they be aware of it next time?) and to compare autopsy reports with physicians' diagnoses (did errors or incompetence contribute to the death?). Another safeguard in a modern hospital is the so-called tissue committee, which reviews pathology reports to see whether the appendix that the surgeon removed was actually diseased, or the tumor excised was malignant. Such procedures sometimes fail, but they do not exist at all either in Zimbabwe's overtaxed public hospitals or in profit-making clinics such as Avenues.

Just how urgent the need is for such oversight became apparent to Charles Khaminwa in the months that followed Lavender's death. He realized from the first that it did not help that he was black while the

---

5. Gerald Bloom, "Two Models for Change in the Health Services in Zimbabwe," *International Journal of Health Services*, Vol. 15 (1985), pp. 451–468.

doctors who treated Lavender were white; yet he had considerable advantages, including postgraduate training in law at Columbia and Cornell and a family income that allowed him to devote full time to the case. Still, Khaminwa and his wife were unable to bring the doctors responsible for Lavender's death to justice—and if he failed, what chance would more ordinary Zimbabwean citizens possibly have in an effort to make medicine accountable?

The Khaminwas' frustrating campaign began on the day of Lavender's death. They waited at the clinic during the surgery, spoke with her briefly in the recovery room, and returned home when visiting hours were over. At 9:00 PM they received a telephone call from the clinic that Lavender had "collapsed"; they rushed back, but by the time they arrived, she was dead. In a state of shock and anger, they went to see the anesthesiologist, Richard McGown, but all he would say was that the child had suddenly stopped breathing. They demanded to talk with the surgeon, who returned to the hospital to meet with them, but he had nothing to add.

They turned next to Avenues Clinic for information, but its administrators refused to provide details about the incident or to order its own investigation. The chief executive officer explained that the clinic was not legally responsible for the physicians' medical practices. "All patients are admitted in the care of their own medical practitioner," he said. "The facilities, equipment and nursing care only are provided by the Clinic." If anything went awry, the doctor and patient had to resolve it between themselves.[6]

This policy of limited responsibility reflected Avenues' determination to return profits to its investors. Its exclusive concern was to get local doctors to use the hospital—the more of them who sent their

---

6. G. Feltoe and T.J. Nyapadi, *Law and Medicine in Zimbabwe* (Harare: Baobab Books in association with the Legal Resources Foundation, 1989), p. 21.

patients to Avenues, the larger its revenues would be. Since some of them would not like the idea of committees to monitor medical practice and the quality of care, the clinic did not provide for any supervision. There were no departmental divisions at Avenues, no chief of medicine or of surgery who might take note of a colleague who consistently made errors. Since the clinic was not affiliated with Harare's medical school, there were no interns or residents to provide emergency treatment, or to observe the quality of care by senior physicians. Since correcting these glaring deficiencies would cost money and limit the physicians' discretion, neither the administrators nor the staff at Avenues were willing to do anything about them.

The Khaminwas managed, after considerable wrangling, to obtain Lavender's hospital chart and to have three doctors of their own choosing present, including one from Kenya and one from South Africa, when the autopsy was performed. From the autopsy they learned two critical facts: that the anesthesia she was given was, to say the least, unorthodox, and that the care that she received in the first hours after the surgery was grossly deficient.

The mix of anesthesia that McGown used to put Lavender to sleep and to keep her asleep during the surgery was standard (nitrous oxide and halothane). But between putting her to sleep and the start of the surgery, he administered, through a spinal injection, four milligrams of morphine. Why he did so remains something of a mystery, for it was wholly unnecessary. The most likely explanation is that a number of anesthesiologists in Europe and in South Africa are using morphine in this way to reduce the stress of surgery in very elderly or high-risk patients, such as those with significant cardiac disease. (The morphine serves as a bridge between the anesthesia during surgery and the painkillers given to the patient later on.)

Apparently McGown had heard about the new technique, was eager to try it, and then did so altogether inappropriately on a healthy ten-year-old. Worse yet, this combination of morphine and anesthesia can suppress both the heart rate and respiration rate, and the condition of anyone receiving it should be checked every fifteen minutes for the first several hours after surgery. But the clinic staff only checked Lavender's condition every hour. Thus she apparently died from respiratory arrest brought on by faulty anesthetic technique and inadequate nursing supervision.

To make a formal complaint, Charles and Mary Khaminwa went to the Health Professions Council, which was set up originally under Rhodesian law to establish the qualifications for doctors and license those who meet them; it also investigates cases of "improper or disgraceful conduct" and "grossly incompetent medical practice," and is empowered to reprimand, fine, and, in the most serious cases, remove from practice those it finds guilty. In October 1990, the Khaminwas asked the council to review Lavender's case and to allow them to present evidence of wrongdoing. The council agreed to investigate but never asked them to testify or to submit evidence (such as the devastating autopsy reports of their experts); it never even permitted them to hear or review the evidence that others submitted. In January 1991, when the Khaminwas asked for a progress report, the council issued the following terse reply: "It is not Council policy to apprise a complainant of the procedures adopted and to issue progress reports. When the investigation is completed you will be advised."

After the Khaminwas made several more inquiries, the head of the council finally agreed to a meeting, which he opened by handing them a letter:

> The Council has now completed its investigation ... and determined there was no negligence or incompetence on the part of the surgeon, the anaesthetist or the nursing staff at the Avenues Clinic.... The anaesthetist followed recognized procedures and the nursing staff carried out their duties in accordance with the doctor's (written) instructions.

As far as the council was concerned, the matter seemed to be closed. If Lavender's parents disagreed with the findings, they were free to bring a malpractice suit in civil court or hope that a police investigation and indictment would lead to prosecution.

Neither course offered much prospect for success. The chief justice of the Supreme Court in Zimbabwe, Anthony Gubbay, told us that he could not recall a single malpractice case in the past twenty years. The international Medical Defense Union, the private group that provides low-cost malpractice insurance worldwide, has observed in a report that Zimbabweans hardly ever consider such an action: "Patients are grateful for the medical attention received and in any case are not litigious."[7]

One reason malpractice suits are rare is that it is illegal for lawyers in Zimbabwe (as in England) to accept a case on a contingency fee. (In the United States, malpractice lawyers sue at their own expense, and take a percentage of the award—generally one third—should they win.) And costs are all the more prohibitive in Zimbabwe, where plaintiffs who win their lawsuit are awarded damages only for lost income and out-of-pocket expenses, not for "pain and suffering." In the case of a child's death, damages are limited to medical and funeral costs, which would amount to much less than attorneys' fees.

The Khaminwas did everything they could to bring the police into the case. Since Lavender died immediately after surgery, the police were required to perform an autopsy and they allowed the Khaminwas to bring in their own experts. The autopsy findings persuaded the police that the case should be treated as a "matter of urgency," but their inquiry, like that of the Health Professions Council, dragged on for months. When Charles and Mary Khaminwa repeatedly asked about the delays, the attorney general reprimanded them for a lack of "restraint."

The reasons for the police inaction became apparent when the

---

7. Garth Hill, "The MDU in Zimbabwe," *International Journal of the Medical Defense Union* (Winter 1987), pp. 8–9.

Khaminwas asked the government itself to launch an investigation. To strengthen their case, they documented other instances of medical incompetence by McGown. Mr. A.'s daughter died during surgery to remove a gallstone; Mrs. Z.'s son suffered irreversible brain damage after surgery for circumcision; and Mrs. C. died after having a tooth extracted. But the Khaminwas could not prove that these were cases of malpractice. Anesthesia, after all, carries a real, if low, risk, and without documented findings from autopsies and morbidity and mortality inquiries by other doctors, it is almost impossible to distinguish between a chance event and the work of an incompetent. A lack of oversight makes it almost impossible to document the need for oversight, which is why the clinic so doggedly resisted impartial inquiries.

To ask for a government inquiry put the Khaminwas at some personal risk, since Mugabe has repeatedly demonstrated he will not tolerate even mild challenges to his rule. Although he has never officially proclaimed Zimbabwe to be a one-party state, this appears to be his ultimate goal. He controls the major daily newspapers and radio stations and the Central Intelligence Organization, whose agents are everywhere.[8] During our visit, we were told both by human rights activists as well as prominent doctors that one is well advised to keep silent in Zimbabwe. We had an exceptionally candid interview with one distinguished Harare physician, but he took us out of his comfortable office and talked with us for nearly an hour in a hallway by an open window, away from wiretaps and hidden microphones.

Mugabe made clear his general disdain for political rights the week before we arrived, when the Commonwealth nations met in Harare. Human rights were prominent on the agenda, and Mugabe's opening remarks paid lip service to the Commonwealth's basic principles. But when students at the University of Zimbabwe in Harare were planning to demonstrate at the conference on behalf of free speech, Mugabe

---

8. Carver, "Zimbabwe: A Break with the Past?," p. 90.

sent riot police who stormed the campus and fired tear gas to break up the meeting.[9]

Notwithstanding the repressive atmosphere, the Khaminwas told a group of politically active students at the university about the death of Lavender, and on November 10, 1990, some two hundred of them (including many members of Zimbabwe's most notable human rights organization, the Catholic Commission for Justice and Peace) marched on Avenues Clinic and the Health Professions Council. Linking Lavender's case to their longstanding campaign for free speech and government accountability, they distributed leaflets protesting the "conspiracy of silence" that surrounded Lavender's death. Ten days later they petitioned the attorney general to expedite the police inquiry, only to be told that an investigation was under way and results would be forthcoming.

The demonstration got the attention of some members of Parliament, and one of them introduced a resolution to conduct "a public inquiry into the activities of some doctors at certain private clinics with the aim of bringing the same to book for any malpractice." In the debate, Mugabe's minister of health, Dr. Timothy Stamps, successfully opposed the motion, saying it was not in Zimbabwe's national interests to have an inquiry. Dr. Stamps himself is a very popular figure in Zimbabwe, mostly because he helped to persuade Mugabe to lift the censorship that his government had earlier imposed on all matters relating to AIDS.

Stamps took the opposite approach with the death of Lavender. He praised Avenues for providing high-quality health care at no cost to the taxpayer and insisted that the combination of anesthesia and morphine administered to Lavender was "conventional, safe, and time honoured ... widely used world-wide in many tertiary units." (He

---

9. Angela P. Cheater, "The University of Zimbabwe: University, National University, State University, or Party University?," *African Affairs*, Vol. 90 (1991), pp. 189–205.

disingenuously said that "open heart surgery would be impossible without...this procedure," ignoring that this case involved routine surgery on a healthy child.) Stamps also sought to stifle the press; he criticized one newspaper's coverage of the case as "inappropriate and unacceptable" because it was "not consistent with good public order," and appealed to national pride, noting that Lavender's doctors and anesthesiologist were "respected specialists whose loyalty to Zimbabwe is unquestionable."

But Stamps, in covering up for his colleagues' misdeeds, revealed that he was particularly troubled by the "deliberate assault on [the] Government's attempts to attract and retain competent specialists at terms much less favourable than they could attract just across the border." The kind of investigation demanded by the Khaminwas, he said, would accelerate the physician "brain drain," causing more Zimbabwean doctors to emigrate to Botswana or, increasingly, to South Africa.

This fear was by no means groundless. Physicians have skills that enable them to choose how and where they work. When they become dissatisfied with conditions in one country they can migrate elsewhere —and often do. It is often said, for example, that both the British National Health Service and American inner-city hospitals would collapse were it not for the presence of Indian doctors. In Zimbabwe itself the number of doctors declined from 1,733 in 1983 to 1,243 in 1987—the last year for which figures were available when we visited—and the drop occurred despite the fact some sixty physicians a year graduated from Harare's medical school.[10]

Because the government was reluctant to hold doctors accountable for their actions, it failed to set up a more equitable system of health care in the early 1980s. Three quarters of Zimbabwe's population live in rural areas, but for reasons of personal comfort, income, and

---

10. *The Zimbabwe Statistical Yearbook*, 1989, pp. 26–34.

prestige, three quarters of all the physicians practice in the two major cities, Harare and Bulawayo. When the ministry of health announced that new graduates from Harare's medical school would have to serve for five years in rural areas, many of the graduates simply left the country rather than fulfill the obligation. When the ministry responded by cutting the service requirement to two years, that compromise only provoked a strike and failed to stop the doctors from emigrating. The plan was abandoned.

Although everyone could see that many physicians neglect public patients in order to treat paying private patients, neither the Ministry of Health nor the medical establishment was willing to do anything about it. Government salaries and payments to doctors, we were told, were too low to sustain the standard of living they now expect—a house, a car, and private schools for their children. Instead of trying to improve the quality of public medicine—through higher salaries and better equipment, for example—the government simply pointed to the danger of doctors leaving the country if any changes were made.

By persevering in their case, the Khaminwas produced a remarkably revealing account of what happens when a government coddles the medical profession and is unwilling to insist on procedures that will protect patients from harm. The record is oddly reminiscent of the situation we uncovered in an inquiry we made into mistreatment of children in Romania—with a difference.[11]

When we investigated the AIDS epidemic among Romania's orphaned children, we learned how the state can corrupt the profession through excessive interference. Ceauşescu's "pronatalist" policies were aimed at forcing women to have children, and they imposed strict rules of censorship on the medical profession. Ceauşescu ordered doctors to register the names of factory employees who were

---

11. See Chapter 8.

pregnant, and he prohibited discussion of any aspects of AIDS. When physicians followed his orders, violating the Hippocratic oath to respect patient confidentiality and to do no harm, the result was a public health disaster. In Zimbabwe, we learned how the state can corrupt the profession through excessive indulgence, leaving medical professionals entirely to their own devices, while the state-chartered medical organizations themselves did nothing to monitor the quality of medical treatment. The result was also a public health disaster, one that affected both the most vulnerable members of society and the more privileged citizens who use private clinics such as Avenues.

The Zimbabwean experience shows that when free-market economics provides the only controls on medicine, the quality of health care deteriorates. Patients on the public wards and private patients will suffer, the first from lack of care, the others from incompetent care. Zimbabwe's doctors, both at Avenues or on the Health Professions Council, might have compensated for the lack of state regulation by setting up their own review committees. Their failure to do so shows the destructive effect that financial self-interest can have on professional standards.

Postscript

The lessons that emerge from Zimbabwe are all the more important since several other countries, most notably South Africa, have followed the same pattern. No sooner did South Africa begin to throw off its legacy of apartheid and desegregate its health care facilities than whites rushed to establish and rely on private, for-profit clinics. By one calculation, in the 1970s, 30 percent of all health care expenditures went to the 20 percent of the population that had private insurance. Now the figures are 60 percent going to the fortunate 18 percent. Earlier, 40 percent of physicians worked in the private sector;

now the figure is 66 percent.[12] And all the while, there is a notable flight of physicians from South Africa. To date, the countries on the receiving end of the brain drain have done nothing to stop the flow.

As for the resolution of the case of Lavender, in 1995 the anesthesiologist, Richard McGown, was charged with five counts of homicide in the deaths of five patients under his care, including Lavender and a twenty-month-old boy who had undergone routine circumcision. McGown was convicted on two counts—Lavender and the boy—and was sentenced to a year in prison with six months suspended. He appealed the sentence, lost, and then served four of the six months before being released and returned to Scotland. Once there, he was the subject of an inquiry before the General Medical Council of the British Medical Association. In 2002, the council decertified him and struck him off the medical register.

As for Avenues Clinic, it is the hospital that the American embassy recommends today for US citizens who require hospitalization in Harare.

12. Solomon R. Benatar, "Health Care Reform and the Crisis of HIV and AIDS in South Africa," *New England Journal of Medicine*, Vol. 35 (2004), pp. 81–92.

8

AIDS AND ROMANIA'S ORPHANS

AMONG THE FIRST stories about AIDS in underdeveloped countries to capture widespread international attention was the plight of Romania's orphans under the brutal regime of Nicolae Ceauşescu. When Ceauşescu was overthrown in December 1989, a country that had been almost entirely sealed off from communication with the West was suddenly thrown open. Initial reports contrasted Romania's pervasive poverty with the opulent palaces that Ceauşescu had built for himself. But within a few months, European journalists and social workers from aid organizations were uncovering an even worse story: hundreds of infants and children living in state orphan asylums had been stricken with AIDS, and the cadaverous images of these babies were as shocking as the photographs of Nazi concentration camp victims after liberation. The awfulness of the AIDS epidemic was a grisly legacy of the Ceauşescu regime and at the same time raised a puzzling question: How had AIDS infiltrated Romanian orphanages? The country, after all, had been closed, its official policies had been hostile, to say the least, to homosexuals, and there had been little intravenous drug use, because of high cost and low supply. Although there was much yet to learn at that time about the transmission of the AIDS virus, enough was already known to make the epidemic seem odd—indeed, really inexplicable.

A few years earlier, the two of us had moved north, going from the Arts and Sciences division at Columbia's Morningside Heights campus to the medical school in Washington Heights. The change gave us a special status with human rights activists. Through the 1980s, indeed, through the 1990s, their organizations were dominated by lawyers who had little knowledge of or familiarity with medical issues. When one or another health-related problem arose, they would contact us to seek advice. In this way, we were first alerted to the phenomenon of organ trafficking (see Chapter 1). And in this way, we were alerted to the puzzle of AIDS in Romanian orphanages. Shortly after Ceauşescu's removal, Aryeh Neier, then head of Human Rights Watch, asked us to investigate the question of AIDS in those institutions; although his request was unexpected, we were intrigued by his suggestion that there was likely to be a link between Ceauşescu's dictatorial rule and HIV transmission. A few weeks later, in June 1990, we went to Bucharest.

The investigation was not difficult to conduct.[1] Orphanage directors and hospital physicians were not averse to being interviewed by visitors from abroad and had no objections to their scrutinizing places that had been hidden away for so long. So, too, officials of the new National Salvation Front government readily discussed (if at times self-servingly) the past record. The health consequences of Ceauşescu's systematically oppressive rule over a country that lacked both democratic traditions and independent associations of professionals, such as doctors, came sharply into view. We were able to understand how a society in which families, not strangers, traditionally cared for the young and the old could produce thousands of abandoned children, and how in a country whose isolation and poverty might have insulated it from HIV, children became part of the AIDS epidemic.

---

1. We were joined in our interviews by Holly Cartner, staff counsel for Helsinki Watch.

*   *   *

In 1990, 683 Romanian children between the ages of one and four had contracted AIDS and at least another 1,000 were HIV-positive. Almost all of them lived in Dickensian institutions where visitors would seldom see a child with a book or toy in hand. This egregious neglect was the product not only of poor oversight and inattention (as is often true in developed countries) but also of deliberate government policies. The orphanages were a desperate attempt by the Ceauşescu government to deal with the consequences of its determination to raise the country's low birth rate. Ceauşescu, by all accounts, was a simpleminded and doctrinaire Marxist, who made production the goal of the state and classified citizens by their productive capacities. In October 1966, one year after taking power, he issued "pronatalist" laws aimed to compel women to bear children. (In 1965, there were only six thousand more births than deaths.) He banned all forms of contraception, increased taxes on childless couples, and, most important, prohibited abortion. In Romania, as in Eastern Europe and the Soviet Union, birth control pills, condoms, and IUDs were scarce and expensive, and abortion was the primary means of contraception. In 1965 approximately one million abortions are estimated to have been performed in Romania, terminating 80 percent of all pregnancies.[2]

The immediate impact of Ceauşescu's pronatalist policies was to increase population growth, which rose to a rate of 18 per 1,000 in 1967. But couples found a variety of ways to avoid having children (such as using the rhythm method and frequenting prostitutes), and the numbers began to go down (in 1975 to 10.4 per 1,000, and in 1980, 7.6). During the 1980s births fell by 2.9 per 1,000, during a time of severe economic stagnation and desperate hardship (exacerbated by

---

2. See Mary Ellen Fischer, *Nicolae Ceauşescu: A Study in Political Leadership* (Lynne Rienner, 1989), particularly Chapter 7; John Hale, *Ceauşescu's Romania* (George Harrup, 1971), p. 142; and Robin Morgan, *Sisterhood Is Global* (Anchor Press, 1984), p. 578.

Ceauşescu's determination to pay off all foreign debt), which gave Romania the lowest per capita income of any European country.[3]

The regime's response was to intensify its policies for promoting more births. To qualify for a legal abortion, a woman now had to have five, as opposed to four, children at home under the age of eighteen. But it was all stick, no carrot. Ceauşescu did not try to make things easier for families with children: maternity leaves were the briefest in Eastern Europe, large families received few tax benefits, and day care and kindergarten services were utterly inadequate.

From the start, the regime conscripted the medical profession into its pronatalist campaign. Gynecologists were required to conduct periodic examinations of women (every four months at factories, for example) and to register the names of all those who were pregnant; they were prohibited from fitting women with IUDs and were required to report anyone coming to a hospital with complications from attempted abortions. On the whole, enough doctors cooperated with the regime that the denials of complicity we often heard rang hollow, and even those denials went only so far. No physician we met admitted to having performed abortions, but they all said they knew of someone who had—perhaps for reasons of principle, more likely for money. A few of these physicians had been caught, tried, and jailed for terms of two to three years. Had the medical profession and its leading members ever taken a stand against the gynecological examinations, we asked, or, for that matter, had they criticized any of Ceauşescu's other brutal medical and social policies? Not that anyone could recall.

Which groups in the population were most affected by the policy of promoting births? Not the urban middle class, whose members managed to obtain contraceptives on the black market—the preference being for an IUD if a doctor could be bribed to fit it. They could

---

3. Michael Shafir, *Romania: Politics, Economics and Society* (London: Francis Pinter, 1985), pp. 127–128.

also afford medical abortions: a Bucharest student told us that several years ago when his girlfriend became pregnant, the abortion had cost him 5,000 lei (about $50 on the black market). And several women with professional degrees told us matter-of-factly that when the government gynecologist-inspector had come to their offices to examine the female staff, they had simply refused to cooperate, and nothing more was heard about it. Nor were most of the people in the more rural parts of the country deeply affected. Those who were devout Christians had long shunned birth control and abortion, and others, like the Gypsies, chose not to practice it.

The brunt of the policy fell on the lower middle class, particularly factory workers, single women, urban Gypsies, and those from disorganized or troubled families, none of whom had the cash or the connections to circumvent the regulations. The choices open to women were as limited as they were threatening to their lives. Some of the women used dangerous methods to carry out abortions by themselves; others went to cheap back-alley abortionists or carried their babies to term, and some may have turned to infanticide.

The exact numbers will never be known, but every physician we spoke to reported that deaths of women from septicemia had been frequent during the Ceauşescu years; abortion-related deaths may have increased by as much as 600 percent after 1966.[4] Indeed, many physicians were certain that botched abortions also accounted for a significant number of birth defects and handicaps. (This was not the only cause: the toxic conditions in workplaces were probably more damaging.)

One point is indisputable: during the 1970s and 1980s, the number of unwanted children increased dramatically. Some women gave birth and abandoned the infants immediately. Others took them home and when they did not have the money to feed them, brought

---

4. Morgan, *Sisterhood Is Global*, p. 578.

them back to the hospital malnourished and abandoned them there. As the director of one orphanage put it, every child has its own story, but virtually every story opens with Ceauşescu's pronatalism.

The regime's response was not to modify its edicts but to create a network of custodial and caretaker institutions that might, at first, seem reasonably conceived but in fact was bizarre and cruel. At the base of the system, serving all children between birth and three years old, were the *leagane*, as orphanages for the very young were called, with a total of 11,000 to 15,000 residents, under the administration of the Health Ministry. Children considered physically and mentally "normal" went on from there to institutions that housed three- to six-year-olds, and then to those that served six- to eighteen-year-olds. Some 40,000 children between three and eighteen were under the jurisdiction of the Education Ministry in these institutions.

Children found to be abnormal, that is, those that a team of psychologists and pediatricians diagnosed as "irrecuperable" because of physical or mental disability, were consigned to separate institutions. Those for children aged three to eighteen held 15,000 residents; the institutions for young people eighteen and over held another 15,000. By an odd leap of logic, a regime that prized productivity assigned the care of these children, classified as "unproductive," to the Ministry of Works. But to this ministry, of course, these children were of little importance. Officials had no interest in their problems and no skills to assist them. No one was motivated or trained to organize rehabilitation or educational services or to establish therapeutic programs for disabled children.

Not surprisingly, conditions in the orphanages for normal children administered by the Education Ministry were not as grim as those in the institutions for the handicapped. In fact, a few of the orphanages, such as Leaganu Number 1 in Bucharest, had been showpieces for the regime, not only to fend off foreign criticism but to attract foreign capital: just as Ceauşescu was willing to send Jews to Israel and

Germans to Germany if he was paid the right price, he also sold orphans to would-be parents. They came to Leaganu Number 1, saw the child, paid hard currency (anywhere from $1,000 and up), and took home a white baby. Thus a policy initiated to increase the national birth rate culminated in the selling of thousands of infants—just how many we probably will never know.

However coercive Ceauşescu's pronatalism and however wretched most of the institutions, the question remains why, as of 1990, 683 children between the ages of one and four had contracted AIDS, and how at least another 1,000 were HIV-positive. The immediate cause of the epidemic, to use the technical term, was nosocomial—HIV infection was conveyed through medical treatment. The political and economic practices of the Ceauşescu regime helped create the conditions in which the disease could spread. And then Romanian doctors and nurses, through ignorance, incompetence, cowardice, and frustration, were responsible for spreading it.

The regime systematically subverted the professionalism of medicine. It isolated physicians from colleagues abroad and from each other at home. By constantly hoarding foreign currencies, the government made it nearly impossible for libraries or doctors to subscribe to foreign journals, obtain foreign books and reports, or travel to conferences. (A kind of medical samizdat did exist, with cigarettes bartered for copies of important articles, but most scientific publications were generally unavailable.) This intellectual quarantine guaranteed that Romanian medicine would be a backwater, even as it was training many third-world doctors (since Ceauşescu wanted their hard-currency payments).

With even graver consequences, the regime refused to acknowledge the presence of AIDS and went so far as to prevent information about the disease from circulating among physicians. As late as 1989, medical meetings could not include a session on AIDS. The most damaging result of that policy was that no attempt was made to screen the blood supply. By 1985, the technology for screening was widely in use elsewhere, but not in Romania. The failure to screen blood had devastating consequences, for the epidemic among the children, as we shall see, did not begin until well into 1988. In effect, the outbreak of AIDS among Romania's institutionalized children was not a cruel accident of fate, a regrettable but unforeseeable contingency, but the result of Ceauşescu's determination to conceal the problem of AIDS and to devote no resources to preventing its spread.

To most experts following the pattern of the disease in the West, the risks of an epidemic in Romania would have seemed low. The country was too poor to support an active drug trade, and the regime was so repressive of homosexuality that there was no active gay community through which the disease could spread. Moreover, Romanians rarely went abroad, and aside from some third-world medical students and dock workers, foreigners rarely visited. The cases that appeared in sailors, homosexuals, and foreign students during the mid-1980s might have remained no more than an isolated handful, if not for the fact that some of them donated blood.

Blood was a form of baksheesh in Romania, donated by people who expected to receive favors from the government by doing so. As Dr. André Combiescu, who had just become director of Bucharest's most important medical research institute, informed us, the regime did not coerce people to donate blood but set quotas for various regional offices. The official rate of exchange for every donation was a free meal or one or two days off from work. (When we said that two days' holiday seemed a lot, he remarked that in Ceauşescu's Romania no one worked very hard in the first place.) Unofficially a blood donation might bring a driver's license, or the renewal of a student visa, or a job. So ordinary citizens, foreign students, and workers, including dock workers, had a variety of reasons to donate blood. Most of those who were HIV-positive had not been tested for the virus, and they donated blood along with the rest.

Even with the censorship of medical information and the extorted donations, Romania might still have avoided an epidemic, for in a country where medical technology was relatively primitive, transfusions were rare. There were no bypass operations or hip replacements. (Getting an X-ray, one doctor told us, was like going to Chernobyl.) But it did have the oddest of medical institutions, the dystrophic hospital, which to the best of our knowledge was not to be found anywhere else.

Dystrophic hospitals, as Dr. Combiescu explained, were an ad hoc response in the early 1980s to the regime's insistence, as part of its intensified pronatal campaign, that any death of a child under the age of one had to be the subject of a formal investigation. Not surprisingly, Romanian doctors did everything possible to get infants past their first birthday and, to this end, began to group together all the infants whose lives seemed at risk. By 1989, the so-called dystrophic wards and hospitals for very sick children held some 2,400 patients.

Even in these wards and hospitals, treatment options were very limited. Malnutrition, infections, and anemia were constant threats. The one available intervention was antibiotics and doctors relied on them heavily, which in itself would not have been disastrous, except for the fact that the doctors always insisted on injecting them rather than administering them orally. In third-world countries it is commonplace for patients to demand injections (of whatever sort). Syrups are the lowest order of medication, pills come next, and, at the top, injections. Romanian physicians themselves succumbed to the mania for injections, even though they knew that nurses would administer them without sterilizing the needles. Since hepatitis B was widespread in Romania, many doctors must have realized that it was transmitted through infected needles. Did the nurses themselves know how dangerous their actions were? Perhaps not, for many of them had no formal education beyond two years of high school—the regime refused to invest in nursing courses—and very little on-the-job training. The nurses were often working in unsupervised wards and, to make matters worse, disposable needles were not generally available. Moreover, the containers for sterilizing instruments were antiquated, and nurses were evidently too ignorant or too tired to spend the fifteen minutes necessary to boil the needles.

One last piece must be added to the puzzle: the dystrophic hospitals' methods for treating children included an odd practice called microtransfusion—transfusion of three to six tablespoons of whole blood. The precise origins of the practice are obscure. It may have been a carryover from folk medicine. One American physician told of observing such transfusions in Korea in the 1950s, and another had heard of a similar procedure being used in Eastern Europe before World War II. More likely, the Romanian practice underscores the danger of a little learning: doctors thought that the transfused blood would be rich in proteins, hemoglobin, and antibodies and would boost a weakened infant's immunological system and nutritional state. But as any adequately trained pediatrician knows, it doesn't work that way. Microtransfusions are entirely useless: too few antibodies are transmitted, iron and other nutrients will not be absorbed, etc. The alternative, of course, was to try to feed the children preparations of powdered milk and fats, either orally or intravenously, although if the case were very severe, such interventions might not succeed either. But rather than recognize their limits—respecting medicine's most ancient maxim to do no harm—and subject themselves to questions, forms, and state investigations, Romanian doctors practiced an outlandish form of medicine, and did far more harm than good.

Some infants were sturdy enough to survive their stay in the dystrophic hospitals, and those who were abandoned by their families went to the orphanages. Staff physicians there would also administer microtransfusions and even more often—apparently quite routinely —treat any and all ailments by injecting the children with antibiotics. Apetrie Roxanna, an epidemiologist at the Health Ministry, who had reviewed the hospital treatment charts of AIDS babies in two Romanian provinces, Constanta (150 cases) and Ialomita (100), told us that 120 injections over a four-week period were not uncommon for children in the dystrophic hospitals and in the orphanages. (To her dismay, she reported that the practice was continuing even in the post-Ceauşescu era and she still found notations of microtransfusions on patients' charts.)

Thus, the factors promoting the transmission of HIV all came together in a deadly sequence. Microtransfusions of AIDS-positive blood infected a small number of babies in a dystrophic hospital; needles were reused for administering antibiotics and spread the infection to other patients. When some of these infected infants entered an orphanage and eventually received injections of antibiotics, the reused needles spread the HIV infection to still others in the orphanage. The result was that as of June 30, 1990, the total number of AIDS cases in Romania was 741, of whom 683 were children under four years of age. Although not all mothers of AIDS babies could be identified and tested, it appears that the disease was transmitted from mother to child in fewer than 5 percent of the cases.

What happened to these AIDS babies could easily have been avoided. Twenty-five percent of the cases were diagnosed in 1989, 70 percent between January and June 1990. This fact, together with the high incidence of the disease in infants under four and the likelihood that about one year elapses between the infection of the children and their first symptoms, made it evident that the spread of the disease to children occurred after 1985, and most of it happened after 1988. This plague was truly man-made. Its origins were in Ceauşescu's policies, and it spread because of bad medical practices.

Shortly after coming to power, the National Salvation Front abolished pronatalism, and thousands of abortions were performed daily in Romanian hospitals. Other means of contraception also became available. The number of children in the orphanages declined, in part because admissions were down, but in part, too, because adoptions went up. White babies available for adoption are scarce in both Western Europe and the United States, and would-be parents flocked to Romania to find them; not surprisingly, no one in the Health Ministry supervised the adoption process closely or tried to keep the babies in the country. Most notably, many European and some American organizations, as well as hundreds of foreign private citizens, came to Romania to provide care to children in practically every institution and hospital in Romania and to provide technical assistance to the Romanian staff.

We ended our first visit with a keen sense that these changes notwithstanding, the heritage of the Ceauşescu regime would be difficult to overcome. Even professionals in Romania had an ingrained suspicion of practically everything they heard or read, particularly if it came from official circles. Having been subjected to doublespeak, lies, and rumors for so many years, they had difficulty distinguishing fact from propaganda. So the microtransfusions continued, as did the cult of injections, despite directives from the Health Ministry and repeated admonitions from visiting doctors and nurses.

Moreover, in view of the poverty and industrial backwardness of the country, we recognized that a number of disasters could occur when the contributions from abroad slackened. Equipment for screening blood for HIV was arriving, but where would the replacement parts come from a year later? The millions of disposable needles that had been sent would last no longer than six months. The lethargy of the workforce was striking, and we were told that some 600,000 Romanians (apparently the ambitious ones) had already emigrated. Who would be left to build the new system of production and distribution that must form the basis of an effective health care and child care system?

With these questions in mind, we met with Dr. Bogdan Marinescu, the new minister of health, who was trained as a gynecologist. A man brimming with energy, he had no illusions about the difficulty of his task or the number of people looking over his shoulder. Although he had been in office only a few months, Dr. Marinescu seemed to have an acute sense of the problems of the system, but little grasp of the limits of his own authority. He was surprised to learn, for instance, that several of his orders—including an order to stop giving microtransfusions and an order to move healthy abandoned children immediately from dystrophic hospitals to orphanages—were disregarded by many institutions. He jotted down names and places. He described the bureaucratic maneuvers he was using to move the institutions for the "handicapped" from the authority of the Ministry of Works to his own.

We raised a troubling issue that came up in many of our talks: since an unknown number of institutionalized children were HIV-positive, and not all of them were clinically ill, was it possible that some would move on to orphanages for three- to six-year-olds and spread the infection further? Dr. Marinescu believed that disposable needles and training would reduce this danger. Clearly someone who respects human rights, he was firmly opposed to the segregation of HIV-positive children in separate institutions.

Dr. Marinescu recognized that sooner or later the numbers of outside helpers would decline, although when we saw him in August 1990 he did not have enough orphanages to fulfill the requests of foreign groups to be assigned entire buildings in which to work. He was working with other officials to persuade foreign companies to open factories in Romania to manufacture IUDs and disposable needles. Dr. Marinescu was acutely aware that economic development would ultimately determine the level of health care, and that unless Romania began to produce a variety of salable goods, it would never be able to sustain an adequate system.

It remained unclear to us whether a government that in June 1990 summoned miners not only to violently attack demonstrations but to terrorize the population generally would be willing or able to deal with the problems we found. Even the limited progress that we observed could have been transitory; the newly appointed heads of the medical institutes and ministries committed to change could be replaced as quickly as they arrived.

In the end, we found it difficult to be very optimistic about the future when the fragility of the Romanian social as well as political order was so apparent. To give adequate health care and child care would require not only substantial resources and efficient monitoring procedures but a degree of professional integrity and discipline in the medical profession that was still notably absent. It was far easier for Ceauşescu to degrade the medical profession than it would be for a new government to rebuild it. And without both a sense of mutual responsibility and discipline, and a system for collegial oversight and censure, physicians, we believed, might well continue their peculiar and dangerous practices. The Romanian experience demonstrated to us that medicine, too, is a liberal discipline and that it depends as much as any other, if not more so, on freedom of expression and respect for the people it treats.

In light of these many questions, we welcomed the chance to return to Romania in 1993, again at the request of Human Rights Watch, to see what had happened in the intervening years. What was the condition of the institutionalized children and the current state of the medical profession? Did the international relief efforts make a difference?

The first thing we learned was that international organizations changed conditions in Romania in a most unexpected way. Hospitals and homes for AIDS orphans and handicapped children had both larger staffs and larger supplies of drugs and equipment than the regular day-care centers and health clinics. The attention given to the children with AIDS helped to remedy shameful conditions, but it also created new problems.

The generous contributions that began in January 1990 had continued and the many relief groups working in Romania were remarkably energetic and enthusiastic. The official Romanian directory of foreign humanitarian organizations working in the country was fifteen pages long and listed 170 groups. Every orphanage had a foreign sponsor, and several Romanian officials wondered whether they should establish a few more institutions so that every interested organization could adopt one. Among the organizations involved were the London-based Romanian Orphanage Trust; the Swedish Save the Children; and the French, Belgium, Luxembourg, and Switzerland chapters of Médecins Sans Frontières. The World Health Organization and UNICEF were active, along with some twenty American organizations, including Project Hope, Project Concern, and Feed the Children. In addition, Princess Margaret, the daughter of Michael, the last king of Romania, had established a foundation devoted exclusively to AIDS babies.

As a result of all this activity, physical conditions in the orphanages we visited in and around Bucharest and Braçov, some two hundred miles to the north, were vastly improved. In Tatarai, where three years earlier we had seen children in rags lying tethered on the bare ground, we now found them decently dressed and playing among the ramps and slides of a modern playground. In 1990, these children had desperately grabbed at us, hungry for human contact and recognition. This time they ignored us and seemed more content. In Mures, the orphanage had the latest in physical therapy devices, and was well stocked with drugs. Almost everywhere we went, we found screened windows, comfortable beds with thick mattresses, colorful plastic dishes and utensils, stalls for showers, hot water, and toilets that flushed.

While these improvements were being made, the number of children in the orphanages dropped by 50 percent. We rarely found two children to a bed, as could be the case in the intensive care units of Romania's general hospitals. The decline partly reflected the impact of legalized abortion. Since the pill and IUDs were not available or were too expensive for 99 percent of the population, abortion remained the primary method of birth control. A country with a population of 22 million had between 800,000 and 900,000 abortions annually. But whatever the psychological effects of frequent abortions, the rates of illness and mortality among Romanian women had declined and there were far fewer abandoned children.

The decline in the numbers of children in institutions also reflected the large number of Europeans and Americans who flocked to Romania to adopt babies, more or less legally from the orphanages, and illegally directly from mothers whom they paid for their babies. By September 1991, Americans alone had adopted some 2,200 Romanian children. (Friday afternoon flights out of Bucharest, we were told, had so many infants on board that companies making baby products were competing to distribute samples to the passengers.) Initially the adopted children came from Romanian orphanages, but when this source was exhausted, a private market in "baby trading" developed, with infants bought directly from their families. By July 1991, so many children were being adopted that with the cooperation of foreign governments, including the United States, Romania declared a ban on private adoptions. (It later reversed the ban and then still later, in light of the sale of babies, reimposed it.)

International organizations also supplied child care institutions with thousands of disposable needles, syringes, and sterilization equipment, along with an ample stock of oral antibiotics and vaccines against hepatitis B. As a result, the spread of both HIV and the hepatitis B virus was markedly reduced. The number of new AIDS cases dropped dramatically; the disease was now found mainly among children between the ages of one and four (1,351 of an estimated total of 1,961), most of whom had been infected during the Ceaușescu years. There seemed to be little infection among adults, but HIV testing was too limited for public health officials to be sure.

Children with AIDS were receiving exceptional medical care. In 1990 the infants we saw at Bucharest's infectious disease hospital, Colintina, were so gaunt and wasted that they resembled concentration camp victims; in 1993, we saw plump and lively children who appeared to be healthy. A team of English nurses supervised their care on cheerful wards decorated with bright murals and filled with toys. These nurses even arranged to open a group home for some twenty of the children on the outskirts of Bucharest. The Colintina children were receiving all available treatments, although not AZT.

But however impressive and reassuring these changes, the legacy of the Ceauşescu era was not easily overcome. The foreign nongovernmental relief organizations (NGOs) were free to do as they pleased. No Romanian agency oversaw them, and the special interests of the sponsoring agency were apparent in each orphanage. If an NGO's self-defined mandate was to donate equipment, then the playgrounds and kitchens were exemplary. If it was dedicated to staff training, the nurses were skilled; if it had missionary aims, religious instruction took precedence. Thus in Romania, as in countries like Mozambique and Cambodia, the NGOs, for all their good works, remained apart from the government and did not share responsibility or power with local groups; as outsiders, they tended to create among the Romanian public some hostility toward themselves and toward the children they were helping.

Just as the Romanian government was incapable of controlling the agencies' day-to-day activities, it could not force them to meet their commitments. In 1990, teams from the French-based Architectes du Monde, modeled on Médecins du Monde, came to Bucharest to renovate old buildings and construct new ones. They promised to divide the costs of several proposed building projects, and, taking the group at its word, the government, at considerable expense, began to construct a new building for children with AIDS at Colintina hospital. But Architectes du Monde never made good on its promise and the shell of a half-completed building stood forlornly on the hospital grounds.

The weakness of government supervision also meant that Romanian institutions set their own policies, subject to the wishes of the international agencies. Every orphanage we visited segregated children who were HIV-positive, and no one, so far as we could find, protested this discrimination. The children were quarantined in their own wards and not allowed to play or eat with the others.

Several institutions were reserved exclusively for children with AIDS, such as the eighty-bed facility at Vidra, some fifteen miles outside Bucharest. Thanks to financial and technical help from several European organizations, the institution was well maintained and the director, an energetic pediatrician, seemed deeply committed to the welfare of her charges; during our conversations, children raced in and out of her office, where they were given candy and cookies. But the pernicious influence of a segregated system was also apparent. As the children at Vidra reached school age, the director had to battle to get them enrolled in the local schools. The townspeople, who had always been uneasy about the presence of an AIDS center, wanted to exclude them. In Vidra, as elsewhere, it was not difficult to stigmatize children.

Moreover, the de facto rule of the NGOs made life easy for medical adventurers. In 1992, David Hughes, a sixty-one-year-old Scottish inventor and researcher (with a doctorate in "hyperbaric physiology" from the University of Grenoble), arrived at Colintina Hospital and easily persuaded its director and its staff to let him test his new cure for AIDS on their children. His drug proved worthless and, luckily, harmless. But such casual experiments on children reveal just how vulnerable the system was to abuse.[5]

When we spoke with Dr. André Combiescu, head of Bucharest's most respected medical research and pharmaceutical production institute, he told us how relieved he was not to be bartering cigarettes

---

5. *Nature*, Vol. 347 (1990), p. 606. Hughes also managed to carry out an earlier AIDS trial in Lolongwe, the capital of Malawi.

for xerox copies of medical journal articles and how pleased he was to be sending his best graduate students abroad. Students felt that they were part of an international community of researchers.

Some attempts were also being made to give medicine a much-needed sense of professional ethics. A recently enacted governmental decree on the "Basic Principles of the Status of the Profession" declared that "the physician is not a public functionary," that he has "total professional independence in the interests of the patient's health."[6] (In fact, much of the document's language is lifted almost verbatim from a Helsinki Watch report that we wrote after our first visit.)

The decree demonstrated that some Romanian physicians were listening to outside criticism, but it did not provide means for enforcing the goals of its high-flown language. Romanian medical societies remained weak and disorganized and many doctors were incompetent. Professors of medicine from abroad were often amazed at the ignorance and lack of training of local doctors, including those at the university medical hospitals. We also heard numerous stories about corruption and greed among physicians. Private practice was still outlawed, and official salaries remained very low (below the level of municipal workers). Doctors, particularly specialists like surgeons, insisted that prospective patients pay them under the table, in money or in goods. Patients who couldn't pay found that they were ignored.

People often told us that doctors wanted to be free from state control not to gain autonomy as professionals but for the larger rewards of private practice. Physicians frequently told us that once patients paid them directly, medicine would become more honorable, efficient, and effective. When we suggested that the fee-for-service system in the US was often inequitable and ineffective, they did not want to hear about it.

---

6. *Viata Medicala* (May 13, 1992) reprinted the decree as promulgated on April 30, 1992.

Thanks to international medical and humanitarian agencies, many of the children that Ceauşescu most despised were favored, indeed privileged. As might be expected, the change had produced public resentment. When we traveled about the country, our interpreter, a Bucharest doctor, was at first amazed and then became increasingly angry when she found that drugs were in greater supply and more up-to-date than at her clinic. The staff members were more alert than those working with her own children in public school. So, too, other physicians were dismayed by the differences between the wards for AIDS children and the wards for adults with nonfatal diseases at Colintina Hospital. To walk the hundred yards separating them was to go from first-class to third-class medicine.

Such objections were predictable, but not persuasive. The charitable funds now supporting children with AIDS almost certainly would not have gone to "normal" Romanian children. Moreover the desperate plight of the powerless orphaned children with AIDS or handicaps justified all the outside help they had been given. Because the new initiatives reflected the policies of outside groups, however, and not a Romanian consensus, they risked being reversed. And so questions remained: What would happen when European and American organizations eventually left Romania? Would the country be capable of manufacturing its own needles, syringes, antibiotics, and condoms? Would it be able to adequately promote health and social welfare? Indeed would it pay any attention at all to its most handicapped citizens?

Surprisingly, we found some grounds for optimism. Probably the most promising was the World Bank's decision to give Romania a $150 million loan over fifteen years to reorganize its health care system. In recognizing health care as part of the country's fundamental economic needs, the bank's experts proved informed and perceptive. They allocated funds for medical equipment and supplies to rural, maternal, and child health care clinics, and for training programs for physicians and nurses. The bank also sought to reorganize the Romanian pharmaceutical industry so as to ensure an adequate supply of drugs and vaccines. Finally, the bank underwrote the planning for a new, decentralized health care system that would be more responsive to the patient, and more competitive. Romania is not the only country where the World Bank invested in health care, but it is doubtful that it would have made so large a commitment without the AIDS scandal.

Although Romania's deep political and economic problems remained acute, we found many dramatic changes since 1990. Privatization put money in some people's hands, and Bucharest now had shops, cafés, and restaurants with plenty of customers, while the lines in front of food stores were much shorter. It is true that disparities in income had become greater than ever and that those living on salaries or fixed incomes were worse off than before. But on our previous visit we had found a mood of unrelieved depression; this time many people told us that at least opportunities to set up new businesses were becoming available.

In one of the hospitals we visited, we met with a physician in her early fifties who talked about what it had been like to grow up under Nazi rule and then spend most of her adult life under Ceauşescu's. She told us in detail how heavy the hand of the state had been, and how physicians had willingly followed medically dangerous regulations without doing anything to protect their patients. She was ashamed of her own part in the system that had transmitted AIDS to babies in her hospital. Then in 1990, she saw, miraculously, the children coming back to life, thanks to foreign food, drugs, and clothing, and to the many nurses who had come from abroad to treat them. But the HIV virus would soon take its toll: within a few years, all of the children would be dead. That much was certain. What remained uncertain was whether the country itself could escape a large-scale disaster.

Final Thoughts, 2005

Romania has escaped disaster—that much is clear. The World Bank's most recent Country Brief declared that it is "comprehensively reforming and restructuring its economy with a view to joining the EU in 2007." Although poverty, particularly rural poverty, persists (25 percent of the population falls below the poverty line), it is enjoying "robust GDP growth...while inflation and interest rates decline steadily." Indeed, the World Bank was pleased to note that "Romania is now a visible and attractive destination for international investors."[7] Challenges abound, from reducing barriers to economic growth to reforming the legislative process. But the bank, now Romania's largest creditor, continues to supply it with capital, $486 million in 2003 and $230 million in 2004.

Medicine and the medical profession have undergone some changes, most of them the result of the shift from a state-run to a market system of health care. Physicians are no longer government employees and may open a private office, which some 15 percent of them have done. Many patients are, to a degree at least, covered by a health insurance system that is employer-based; payroll contributions provide most of the funds for health care, although some 30 percent of expenditures are out of pocket. Hospitals, however, remain under state control and are still at the center of the health care system. Overall quality of care is, by most estimates, low, and the profession itself exerts little influence over medical practice or health policy. Romania is still eight years below the EU average for life expectancy (sixty-eight versus seventy-six); its infant mortality rate is three and a half times higher.[8]

---

7. World Bank, Romania Country Brief 2004.

8. European Observatory on Health Systems and Policies, report on Romania, 2000, www .observatory.dnk; Cristan Vladescu, Center for Health Policies and Services, Silviu Radulescu, World Bank, and Victor Olsavsky, WHO liaison officer to Romania.

As for AIDS, we can now better calculate, and deplore, the full effects of the Ceauşescu policies on the orphaned children. In 1989–1990, there were 468 children under one year of age with AIDS. The number then dropped over the ensuing years (in 1991, forty-three, in 1995, eight, in 2004, zero). But over the same years, AIDS moved up the age ladder. In 1989–1990, there were 924 cases among one- to four-year-olds, then 486 cases in 1991, 416 cases in 1992, and 327 in 1993. Only after 1996 did the rate drop off in this cohort—but it then appeared in the five- to nine-year-olds and, subsequently, in the ten- to fourteen-year-olds. The only relief from all this tragedy is the 2004 figures: five cases in children below the age of nine, ten cases in children ten to fourteen.[9] Finally, fifteen years later, the Ceauşescu curse is almost over.

And what, finally, of the orphans and the orphanages? The system is still close to chaos. It does appear that the number of institutionalized children is dropping. Although record-keeping is far too inadequate to allow for firm numbers, the best guess is that some 170,000 children were institutionalized in the early 1990s. The government then began to push a foster care system, and the numbers dropped to around 60,000 in 2001 and to 32,000 today. Conditions in urban facilities have improved but rural ones are still wretched; institutions serving children are better than those serving adults. As a 2005 report to the Open Society Institute explained, deinstitutionalization is now the official government policy but changes will come only very gradually. In the meanwhile, the OSI report found serious overcrowding and "in the worst cases, conditions are inhuman and degrading, clearly violating basic human rights."

Such findings help to make the controversies around international adoption of Romanian children more bitter. As Elisabeth Rosenthal

---

9. The data are drawn from "HIV/AIDS in Romania 1985–2004," reported by the Dr. Matei Bals Infectious Diseases Institute, HIV/AIDS Monitoring and Evaluating Department, under the direction of Dr. Adrian Streinu-Cercel at Carol Davila Medicine University.

reported in June 2005 in *The New York Times*, the EU had demanded in 2002 that Romania reform its child welfare programs, and UNICEF estimates that some 10,000 children are still abandoned every year in the hospitals. The government, desperate to remove barriers to entering the EU, responded by banning the institutionalization of newborns and promoting its family care and foster care programs. It also recommitted itself to a ban on foreign adoptions. Critics charge that foster care programs are too inadequate to resolve the many problems and that adoptions should be allowed. The government says it is rethinking its policy, but it wants to protect the interests of the biological mothers, and worries about a resurgence of baby selling. As of now the ban is in effect and no one is happy.

9

WORKING STIFFS: THE MEDICAL RESIDENT
AND MEDICINE AS A PROFESSION

EXCEPT FOR Karen Ann Quinlan's, no other patient's death has transformed American medical practice as much as that of Libby Zion. Karen Ann Quinlan made history in the mid-1970s when the medical staff at St. Clare's Hospital in New Jersey would not remove her from a respirator, as her parents wished them to do, even though she was in a "persistent vegetative state." The Quinlans took the hospital to court and eventually won their lawsuit on appeal; in doing so they helped to define the ethical standards by which the question of when to take someone off life-support systems is now decided. Libby Zion made history in 1984, when she died eight hours after entering New York Hospital's emergency room with seemingly minor complaints of fever and earache. Her parents, too, took the hospital to court. Even though they did not win their case, they brought into the open the need to reform one of the least well understood aspects of American medicine: its residency training programs.

After years of inquiry into Libby Zion's death no one can be sure why she died, and who, if anyone, was to blame. A grand jury considered bringing criminal charges against her doctors; the state's Professional Medical Conduct Board held extensive hearings, and a civil court gathered testimony in a trial that lasted several months. To this day no one is certain why an apparently healthy eighteen-year-old suddenly developed a fever that soared to a fatal 108 degrees.

One popularly held theory appeared as Question 49 on a pharmacology examination given to second-year students at the Columbia College of Physicians and Surgeons:

> Which of the following drugs was administered in the Zion case at New York Hospital and had an interaction with an antidepressant MAO inhibitor that was fatal?
>
> A. Morphine
> B. Meperidine
> C. Fentanyl
> D. Codeine
> E. Heroin

The correct answer, according to the examiners, was B, meperidine, more commonly known as Demerol. That answer, however, was wrong. It is true that Libby Zion was taking an antidepressant, and that the New York Hospital staff should have known better than to give her a sedative like Demerol. But the dose they gave her was very low (in fact, too low to be effective), and there is no case on record of anyone dying from the two drugs as administered.

Libby's parents also got it wrong. Their major claim (among many others) was that the staff physicians were so exhausted from lack of sleep that they could not treat their daughter properly. Not only did they prescribe Demerol incorrectly, but when the nurse on duty reported that Libby was thrashing about, the intern, instead of going to see her, ordered her tied to her bed. In fact, whatever errors were committed were not the result of fatigue. One of the interns was coming off a weekend break and the other had just begun his shift in the emergency room.

New York Hospital also got it wrong. Its lawyers and spokesmen blamed the patient. Had Libby Zion candidly informed the hospital staff about all the drugs she was taking—more precisely, had she told them that she was using cocaine—the outcome, they said, would have been different. But while there was evidence that Libby had taken cocaine shortly before being admitted to the hospital, it was not conclusive. One postmortem analysis revealed a trace of the drug in her nostrils; a second did not. Indeed, the bungling that surrounded the testing of blood and tissue in the Zion case calls to mind the O. J. Simpson case. In both, medical examiners showed a knack for raising more questions than they could resolve.

Even more important, New York Hospital's effort to shift the blame makes one ask why its doctors had not diagnosed the drug problem themselves. Libby had several textbook symptoms of cocaine use—fever, spastic movements, disorientation—which should have prompted doctors in the emergency room to admit her to intensive care for close observation. But the failure to send Libby to that unit never received the attention it deserved, in or out of court—not the least of the reasons being that the Zions were unwilling to concede that their daughter was likely to have used cocaine. Had they been more open about it, they might have won their case on the grounds that even if their daughter had used cocaine, she still should have had the more careful treatment that would have saved her life.

The various legal and medical groups that reviewed the incident did nothing to clarify the cause of death or to ascertain where the ultimate responsibility for it lay. Not only did a grand jury refuse to indict the doctors on criminal charges, but the state Professional Medical Conduct Board refused to revoke their licenses. The jury in the civil suit brought by the Zions found fault with both sides. It said that the physicians were negligent in prescribing Demerol and that the intern in charge of Libby Zion was negligent in not following her changing condition more closely and not consulting with senior doctors. But it also found that Libby Zion had taken cocaine soon before her death and had herself been negligent in not providing her doctors with a full and accurate medical history. By blaming everyone, the jury left open the question of whether Demerol, cocaine, incompetence, or viral disease had precipitated Zion's death.

Natalie Robins's book *The Girl Who Died Twice*[1] is not able to answer the questions that have eluded so many others. A diligent journalist, Robins provides a thorough, if somewhat disjointed, account of a very complex case. She tracked down Libby's friends, followed the various court hearings assiduously, and spoke to many doctors about medical training in hospitals (although that did not, as we will see, save her from some serious misconceptions about it). Her account moves back and forth between scenes from Libby's life as she grew up and interviews with the doctors who treated her at New York Hospital. As the book's title suggests, to understand the death of Libby Zion one must look into the history both of the Zion family and of New York Hospital.

Libby and her father, Sidney Zion, dominate Robins's account of the family. (She says little about relations between mother and daughter and it is hard to imagine what they were.) Drawing on interviews with Libby's friends and on their court depositions, Robins depicts Libby as a likable but confused and lonely teenager. She missed many classes in high school and at Bennington College. Her relationships with young men were tangled and unhappy. Like many others of her generation, she used drugs, including cocaine and marijuana. (Her letters, which were introduced as evidence, include passages in which she says that her brain is in a state of "confusion...due to increased amounts of a certain powder entering it.") And, more than most of her friends, Libby went to doctors. She consulted at least seven, including an internist, a gynecologist, a pediatrician, a psychiatrist, a

---

1. Delacorte, 1995.

dentist, and two school physicians; she collected prescriptions to combat stomach trouble, sleeplessness, and depression. Her internist's chart, which was incomplete, noted that she was taking or had taken Tagamet (for ulcers), Motrin (for pain relief), Actifed (for allergies), Valium and Dalmane (for anxiety), an antibiotic, two anti-inflammatories, an antihistamine, and an antispasmatic; she was also on Nardil, an antidepressant.

Yet her physicians were either unconcerned about or ignorant of the variety of medicines she was taking. Each of them appears to have treated the specific symptoms Libby reported (in person or on the telephone), but paid considerably less attention to the young woman herself. Like many others, Libby knew how to play the medical system, which is so fragmented into mutually exclusive specialties that she had an easy time getting whatever prescription she wanted.

Sidney Zion, a former columnist for *The New York Times* and later co-owner of a midtown Manhattan steak house, was the main complainant against Libby's doctors. Robins's portrait of him is not sympathetic, although she notes that she has known him for more than twenty-five years and that he helped with her research. She describes him as aggressive, self-centered, and self-promoting. (Many people have never forgiven him for divulging on a late-night radio talk show that it was Daniel Ellsberg who had leaked the Pentagon Papers to *The New York Times*.) And, according to Robins, his eulogy at his daughter's funeral had less to say about her life than about his feelings of indignation at what her doctors had done or failed to do.

Sidney Zion pursued New York Hospital and its doctors with an uncontrolled fury. In his view, they had not committed a regrettable but unavoidable medical error, but outright homicide. "It is my definition of a murder," he told the state Professional Medical Conduct Board. This judgment was malicious and preposterous, but he used it to turn the incident into one of the most effective means for bringing change to American medicine: a scandal.

* * *

Although physicians are reluctant to concede it, during the past twenty years the most significant reforms in medicine have been brought about by outsiders. It was mainly lawyers and journalists who helped to stop medical experimentation on human subjects in the US by exposing, among other abuses, the use of unwitting black men for research on syphilis in Alabama and the use of retarded children for research on hepatitis at the Willowbrook State School in New York. It was the relatives of people close to death who forced hospitals and doctors to ask patients whether or not they wished to be kept alive; they supported their case with surreptitiously taken photographs of chalkboards that, unknown to the patients or their families, coded patients on a scale that went from "do everything" to "do nothing." Patients and their advocates have forced doctors to give far more accurate accounts of their diagnoses. And women patients helped to change the dominant practice of performing mastectomies in breast cancer cases, allowing women to choose from among far less drastic alternatives. While some doctors were important in introducing these changes, the medical profession left to itself would not have initiated or accomplished any of them.

The training of hospital residents has now also been subject to reform. If not for Sidney Zion's relentless pursuit of New York Hospital, the unreasonable demands to which hospital residents had been submitted and their consequences for patients would have remained unmodified. Several prominent doctors have expressed regret that it took Sidney Zion to reveal the defects of medical training in hospitals. "My wish would be," conceded Robert Petersdorf, president of the Association of American Medical Colleges, "that the profession had been more perceptive in recognizing the issue and making appropriate changes in training prior to its becoming a cause célèbre." It was, he said, "unfortunate that long-overdue changes in structuring residency training were not initiated within our own community prior to the serendipitous stimulus of the Zion case."[2] But the profession's inertia persisted for decades.

Residency training is a wilderness that few nonphysicians penetrate. Patients lying sick in a hospital bed rarely inquire of the person with a stethoscope whether he or she is an attending physician, a resident, an intern, or, for that matter, a medical student. (In some institutions, the length of the white coat is the giveaway, but few people know that short jackets identify medical students and knee-length coats "attending physicians," the senior doctors formally in charge of a patient's case.) More important, at least until the publicity around the Zion case, almost no one outside medicine appreciated the contradictions inherent in the residency system and their effects on the lives of residents and patients.

These contradictions start with the definition of a resident's status and tasks. Residents are both advanced students and practitioners: the official term for the three-year resident program is "graduate medical education." In fact, many teaching hospitals have dropped the labels "intern" and "resident" altogether, using instead the terms Post Graduate Year I, II, and III. Interns are in their first postgraduate year after taking their M.D. degree; residents are in their second and third. As graduate students, residents are expected to read widely in the medical literature and to consult regularly with their putative teachers—that is, the attending physicians. But residents are also practitioners, responsible on a day-to-day basis for diagnosing, treating, and monitoring anywhere from ten to thirty very sick patients. In many hospitals, they are also expected to do "scut work": drawing blood, inserting intravenous lines, taking specimens to the lab, and so on.

The two roles do not fit together easily either in theory or in practice. Residents are supposed to be supervised as they care for their

---

2. Robert G. Petersdorf, M.D., "Regulation of Residency Training," *Bulletin of the New York Academy of Medicine* (July–August 1991), p. 330.

patients but not supervised too closely. According to the prevailing view, the only way they can learn to practice medicine is by actively making diagnoses, administering drugs, and performing various other medical procedures. If the process is monopolized by an attending physician, the resident's training will suffer. Accordingly, the guidelines issued by the American Board of Internal Medicine, the certifying body for residency programs, state: "Residents must have continuing responsibility for most of the patients they admit.... Residents must be given the responsibility for decision making and for direct patient care."[3] Supervision is important, but direct experience with patients counts most.

While the official requirements are designed to give residents opportunities to make independent decisions, they have very wide discretion. The result is often what one reform-minded physician has called "resident-run residencies." Residents usually have primary responsibility over ward patients (that is, poor patients paid for mainly by Medicaid), which gives them an opportunity to learn from treating patients who do not have personal doctors or specialists of their own. Senior physicians provide supervision, but only up to a point—they usually appear on the wards each morning for two hours and make the rounds of patients accompanied by residents and medical students; they may do the same for an hour or two in the afternoon if they are particularly diligent; they are very rarely present at night. For their part, residents on the wards are seldom eager to consult with the senior physicians; they want to work through the cases themselves. In most teaching hospitals, to wake a supervisor with a question or to ask him to come to the hospital in the middle of the night would amount to a confession of ineptitude.

This system prompted Michel Foucault to observe that with the rise of scientific medicine, the poor and the rich struck a Faustian

---

3. *Graduate Medical Education Directory*, 1995, pp. 62–63.

bargain. The poor received treatment on the wards, and in return gave their bodies to the service of medical education. The rich benefited from this knowledge, and in return endowed and supported the hospitals. But Foucault was only partly right. Residents learn not only by treating the poor but by caring for private patients as well. Even people who endow hospitals or have their own personal doctors or specialists seldom escape the system. All but a few private patients in teaching hospitals go "on service." That is, they are seen regularly by the resident staff, which writes out their "orders," including the tests and procedures they are to undergo and the medicine they are to be prescribed. Each patient has an "order book" in which his treatment is entered. It is not always officially closed to attending physicians in the sense that they are prohibited from writing in it; but in practice the orders are entered by the residents, both for "on service" patients as well as for ward patients. Indeed, the American Board of Internal Medicine flatly states: "Residents cannot be expected to show appropriate growth in understanding patient care responsibilities if others write orders for patients under the residents' care."

Before Libby Zion's death her family had little idea how a hospital worked. They assumed, for example, that since their doctor had sent Libby to the emergency room at New York Hospital, he would be in charge and on the scene. But the case was handled in the usual way— that is, Libby was put "on service." In fact, the residents called and spoke to the attending physician several times. No record exists of these conversations, but it seems most unlikely from the evidence that the residents told him, or implied, that he should come to the hospital. Neither the admitting diagnosis ("viral syndrome with hysterical symptoms") nor the admitting orders (to merely monitor the patient's vital signs) suggested that Libby's condition was critical. When a nurse asked an intern to see the increasingly agitated patient, the intern treated her request casually, as if there was no cause for intense concern. In those circumstances few private physicians would have gone to the hospital; most of them would have done so only if they had an urgent call from the house staff or if they had a special relationship with the patient.

Would a more experienced doctor have sent Libby to the intensive care unit? Should not the intern have come to see Libby as her fever rose? In hindsight most of the physicians I know would say yes to both questions, but there is no way to be sure what should have been done at the time. All that can be said is that no senior physician on the hospital staff ever examined Libby. Neither New York Hospital nor most other hospitals kept a senior doctor on hand to review decisions made by emergency room residents. That they should now do so was one of the two major proposals for reform that were provoked by Libby Zion's death.

The second and more far-reaching reform concerned how long residents work. Until the Zion case, it was commonplace for residents to be on the job 100 to 120 hours per week and to be on call every third or fourth night (during the 1930s and 1940s, they were on call every second night). Once or twice a week, each resident worked a thirty-six-hour shift (from 7 AM the first day through 7 PM the second day, returning the next morning at 7 AM). The most obvious result was that residents did almost anything to cut down on their nighttime tasks simply to get some sleep. A harrowing account of their working lives was given in 1986 by the sociologist Terry Mizrahi in her book *Getting Rid of Patients*,[4] which described the variety of strategies residents used to avoid a "hit" (their term for a patient admission) or, failing that, to ease their workload. But Mizrahi's book had no effect on medical training.

Although virtually everyone in charge of medical schools and hospitals recognized the drawbacks of a 120-hour week, they not only accepted the arrangement but strongly defended it. Since patients needed "continuity of care," so the argument went, it was better to

---

4. Rutgers University Press, 1986.

have a tired doctor who knew the case than a rested one who had only read the chart. Critical illnesses, it was said, often develop over several twelve-hour periods; so shorter hours would mean that residents would miss a vital training experience. Most important, residents had to learn that medicine was a calling, not a job, and that one's responsibility to one's patients took precedence over all other considerations, including sleep. Put residents on a fixed schedule and they would come to adopt a lax "shift mentality."

None of these propositions, however, was ever actually tested. In a profession that prides itself on rigorous trials for every new drug and procedure, few hospital directors in the pre–Libby Zion period experimented with different schedules or examined charts to see if the theory of twelve-hour periods had any bearing on how illnesses really developed. No one challenged the idea that sleeplessness instilled a professional ethos in interns or wondered why learning how to avoid seeing patients was so important a part of a young physician's education. When the occasional critic noted that, apart from those in military service in wartime (and, some would add, new mothers or writers and editors facing deadlines), no one else regularly worked under conditions of sleep deprivation, the medical community insisted that a different system would be worse by far.

Ironically, the residents who treated Libby were not working on too little sleep. But once the facts of residency training came into the open, demands for change mounted. To the grand jury that reviewed the Libby Zion case, it seemed obvious that if the Federal Aviation Association said that pilots had to have "nine consecutive hours of rest for less than eight hours of scheduled flight time," residents should not be treating patients for thirty-six hours straight. The grand jury also found that interns were not adequately supervised and recommended that hospitals change the prevailing arrangements for overseeing their work.

In response, David Axelrod, then head of the New York State Department of Health, appointed a commission chaired by Professor Bertram

Bell of the Albert Einstein College of Medicine in 1986. After numerous hearings and over strenuous objections from doctors, the Bell Commission recommended several major reforms which were officially adopted in 1989 as Section 405 of the New York State Health Code. The work week of medical interns was not to exceed an average of eighty hours; they were not to work more than twenty-four consecutive hours and were to have one twenty-four-hour period free each week. Every hospital emergency room had to have an attending physician present and on duty, and every hospital had to have an attending physician on call should residents require a consultation. The state provided hospitals with additional funds to defray the added costs of these reforms, including payments to auxiliary workers to do "scut work" and an increase of about 10 percent in the number of residency slots.

New York's precedent did spur a good deal of discussion about residency and even some attempts to lighten the work schedule. But there was little consensus on the value of making these changes. As might be expected, the residents themselves were overwhelmingly in favor of them. Residents in internal medicine at Albert Einstein College of Medicine told researchers that "the regulations had reduced their fatigue on the wards and lessened emotional stress.... They now provided better patient care."[5] Residents in obstetrics and gynecology at the Columbia-Presbyterian Medical Center said that, with no diminution in the quality of patient care, there was "a marked improvement in the quality of their personal lives, the amount of sleep they achieved, and their level of stress."[6]

---

5. Joseph Conigliaro, William Frishman, Eliot Lazar, and Lila Croen, "Internal Medicine Housestaff and...the Impact of New York State Section 405 Regulations...," *Journal of General Internal Medicine*, Vol. 8 (1993), p. 505.

6. Amalia Kelly, Frances Marks, Carolyn Westhoff, and Mortimer Rosen, "The Effect of the New York State Restrictions on Resident Work Hours," *Obstetrics & Gynecology*, Vol. 78 (1991), p. 468.

On the other hand, senior physicians complained bitterly that residents were adopting a shift mentality and that patient care has suffered. If there were a limit on hours worked, residents would leave tests uncompleted and ignore anyone who challenged them when they headed for home. Most residents deny the charge, maintaining that they are not clock-watchers and have not lost their sense of professional responsibility. Most attending physicians say they do not believe them.

Commentators did recognize that contrary to previous practice, Medicare and HMO regulations now required that only people with very serious illnesses be admitted to a hospital. Patients also were remaining in hospitals for much shorter periods, from an average of twelve days in the early 1980s to less than eight days in the mid-1990s, owing to new and more complex technology for diagnosis and treatment as well as to constantly rising costs. So it was one thing to work thirty-six hours when residents only had to read an EKG or listen to a stethoscope. It was quite another when they might be prescribing fast-acting cardiac drugs or performing more intricate and invasive diagnostic procedures, such as inserting a catheter into the heart to measure its output of blood. Nevertheless, it took another decade, and a different set of players, to get New York's regulation adopted throughout the country.

The force for change, once again, came from outside establishment medical circles. A report on patient safety in 2000 from the prestigious Institute of Medicine, which highlighted many problems in the system, gave no attention at all to the issue of residents' work schedules. The next year, the watchdog group Public Citizen petitioned the Occupational Safety and Health Administration to intervene, but OSHA did not respond. Then in November 2001, John Conyers, a congressman from Michigan, introduced a bill to set an eighty-hour week for residents; in June 2002, Jon Corzine from New Jersey introduced a similar bill into the Senate. That same month—actually the day before Corzine's bill—the American Council on Graduate Medical Education (ACGME), which accredits all residency programs, required as of July 1, 2003, an eighty-hour-a-week limit with one day off every seven and no more than every third night on.

The ACGME readily admitted that it was attempting to ward off government action. Paul Friedman, the co-chair of its committee on resident duty hours, conceded that looming federal action "did prod us...on the recommendation." Jordan Cohen, head of the Association of American Colleges, made the same point: it was "philosophically unacceptable for the profession to abrogate its responsibilities." Government intervention would be "an extremely unwelcome turn of events."[7] The American College of Physicians was no less blunt: "The ACP opposes regulation of residents' work hours by individual states or the federal government." As medicine knows full well, the best defense is a good offense.

Although the debate on the merits of the change continues, with some physicians doggedly insisting that hour limits turn the profession into an occupation, the new regulations are being fairly well enforced. Johns Hopkins, whose residency program in medicine is among the most demanding, first tried to ignore the stipulations. But one of its interns blew the whistle, sent an anonymous email to the ACGME, and complained of working 120 hours. The ACGME investigated and put Hopkins on probation with the possibility that its program would be decertified. The publicity that followed gave the ACGME credibility: if it went after Hopkins, it would go after anyone. And with no small measure of concern, Hopkins put its house staff requirements in order and avoided penalties. Most residency programs now police themselves in strong-arm fashion. Let a resident come up against the time limit, and she will be chased out.

---

7. Robert Steinbrook, "The Debate over Residents' Work Hours," *New England Journal of Medicine*, Vol. 347 (2002), pp. 1296–1302.

In the end, do the hours really matter? The answer is an unequivocal yes. A spate of impressive research over these past several years confirms what many suspected: sleeplessness distorts medical decision-making. Investigators have tested residents' ability to correctly read an EKG or, in simulated fashion, to perform a procedure, and they find marked decrease in performance after prolonged wakefulness. The same is true under real-life situations. A team at Boston's Brigham and Women's Hospital meticulously compared residents' performance when they were and were not sleep deprived. The findings were actually scary: a 36 percent increase in "serious medical errors" when sleep deprived. A few technical details illustrate what this means. In one case, the resident was about to tap the wrong lung on a patient with pleurisy; in another, the resident reported that the fluid levels for a patient in heart failure were stable when he was actually in fluid overload; and in still another, the resident wrote a prescription for an intravenous drip at 0.2 when the correct level was 0.02. Luckily, a nurse caught the mistake in time.[8]

So doctors, even young doctors, are no different than truck drivers and airplane pilots. Keep them awake for inordinate periods of time and they may do irreparable harm.

---

8. The studies were carried out by the Harvard Division of Sleep Medicine and published in the *New England Journal of Medicine*, Vol. 305 (October 28, 2004), pp. 1829–1848.